Pain Management for People with Serious Illness in the Context of the Opioid Use Disorder Epidemic

PROCEEDINGS OF A WORKSHOP

Laurene Graig, India Olchefske, and Joe Alper, *Rapporteurs*

Roundtable on Quality Care for People with Serious Illness

Board on Health Care Services

Board on Health Sciences Policy

Health and Medicine Division

The National Academies of
SCIENCES · ENGINEERING · MEDICINE

THE NATIONAL ACADEMIES PRESS
Washington, DC
www.nap.edu

THE NATIONAL ACADEMIES PRESS   500 Fifth Street, NW   Washington, DC 20001

This activity was supported by Aetna Inc., Altarum Institute, American Academy of Hospice and Palliative Medicine, American Cancer Society, American Geriatrics Society, Anthem Inc., Ascension Health, Association of Professional Chaplains, Association of Rehabilitation Nurses, Blue Cross Blue Shield Association, Blue Cross Blue Shield of Massachusetts, Blue Cross and Blue Shield of North Carolina, Bristol-Myers Squibb, The California State University Institute for Palliative Care, Cambia Health Solutions, Cedars-Sinai Health System, Center to Advance Palliative Care, Centers for Medicare & Medicaid Services, Coalition to Transform Advanced Care, Excellus BlueCross BlueShield, Federation of American Hospitals, The Greenwall Foundation, The John A. Hartford Foundation, Hospice and Palliative Nurses Association, Kaiser Permanente, Susan G. Komen, Gordon and Betty Moore Foundation, National Coalition for Hospice and Palliative Care, National Hospice and Palliative Care Organization, National Palliative Care Research Center, National Patient Advocate Foundation, National Quality Forum, The New York Academy of Medicine, Oncology Nursing Society, Patient-Centered Outcomes Research Institute, Social Work Hospice and Palliative Care Network, Supportive Care Coalition, and the National Academy of Medicine. The MAYDAY Fund also provided support for this project. Any opinions, findings, conclusions, or recommendations expressed in this publication do not necessarily reflect the views of any organization or agency that provided support for the project.

International Standard Book Number-13: 978-0-309-49223-2
International Standard Book Number-10: 0-309-49223-8
Digital Object Identifier: https://doi.org/10.17226/25435

Additional copies of this publication are available from the National Academies Press, 500 Fifth Street, NW, Keck 360, Washington, DC 20001; (800) 624-6242 or (202) 334-3313; http://www.nap.edu.

Copyright 2019 by the National Academy of Sciences. All rights reserved.

Printed in the United States of America

Suggested citation: National Academies of Sciences, Engineering, and Medicine. 2019. *Pain management for people with serious illness in the context of the opioid use disorder epidemic: Proceedings of a workshop.* Washington, DC: The National Academies Press. doi: https://doi.org/10.17226/25435.

The National Academies of
SCIENCES · ENGINEERING · MEDICINE

The **National Academy of Sciences** was established in 1863 by an Act of Congress, signed by President Lincoln, as a private, nongovernmental institution to advise the nation on issues related to science and technology. Members are elected by their peers for outstanding contributions to research. Dr. Marcia McNutt is president.

The **National Academy of Engineering** was established in 1964 under the charter of the National Academy of Sciences to bring the practices of engineering to advising the nation. Members are elected by their peers for extraordinary contributions to engineering. Dr. C. D. Mote, Jr., is president.

The **National Academy of Medicine** (formerly the Institute of Medicine) was established in 1970 under the charter of the National Academy of Sciences to advise the nation on medical and health issues. Members are elected by their peers for distinguished contributions to medicine and health. Dr. Victor J. Dzau is president.

The three Academies work together as the **National Academies of Sciences, Engineering, and Medicine** to provide independent, objective analysis and advice to the nation and conduct other activities to solve complex problems and inform public policy decisions. The National Academies also encourage education and research, recognize outstanding contributions to knowledge, and increase public understanding in matters of science, engineering, and medicine.

Learn more about the National Academies of Sciences, Engineering, and Medicine at **www.nationalacademies.org**.

The National Academies of
SCIENCES • ENGINEERING • MEDICINE

Consensus Study Reports published by the National Academies of Sciences, Engineering, and Medicine document the evidence-based consensus on the study's statement of task by an authoring committee of experts. Reports typically include findings, conclusions, and recommendations based on information gathered by the committee and the committee's deliberations. Each report has been subjected to a rigorous and independent peer-review process and it represents the position of the National Academies on the statement of task.

Proceedings published by the National Academies of Sciences, Engineering, and Medicine chronicle the presentations and discussions at a workshop, symposium, or other event convened by the National Academies. The statements and opinions contained in proceedings are those of the participants and are not endorsed by other participants, the planning committee, or the National Academies.

For information about other products and activities of the National Academies, please visit www.nationalacademies.org/about/whatwedo.

PLANNING COMMITTEE FOR A WORKSHOP ON PAIN MANAGEMENT FOR PEOPLE WITH SERIOUS ILLNESS IN THE CONTEXT OF THE OPIOID USE DISORDER EPIDEMIC[1]

ANDREW DREYFUS (*Co-Chair*), President and Chief Executive Officer, Blue Cross Blue Shield of Massachusetts

JAMES A. TULSKY (*Co-Chair*), Chair, Department of Psychosocial Oncology and Palliative Care, Dana-Farber Cancer Institute; Chief, Division of Palliative Medicine, Brigham and Women's Hospital; Professor of Medicine and Co-Director, Center for Palliative Care, Harvard Medical School

PATRICIA A. BOMBA, Vice President and Medical Director, Geriatrics, Excellus BlueCross BlueShield

STEVE CLAUSER, Director, Healthcare Delivery and Disparities Research Program, Patient-Centered Outcomes Research Institute

REBECCA A. KIRCH, Executive Vice President of Healthcare Quality and Value, National Patient Advocate Foundation

JANE LIEBSCHUTZ, Chief, Division of General Internal Medicine, University of Pittsburgh Medical Center Health System, University of Pittsburgh School of Medicine

SALIMAH MEGHANI, Associate Professor of Nursing and Term Chair in Palliative Care, Department of Biobehavioral Health Sciences; Chair, Graduate Group in Nursing; Associate Director, NewCourtland Center for Transitions and Health; Senior Fellow, Leonard Davis Institute of Health Economics, University of Pennsylvania

R. SEAN MORRISON, Director, National Palliative Care Research Center

JUDITH PAICE, Director, Cancer Pain Program, Division of Hematology-Oncology, and Research Professor of Medicine, Feinberg School of Medicine, Northwestern University

PHILIP A. PIZZO, Founding Director, Stanford Distinguished Careers Institute; Former Dean and David and Susan Heckerman Professor of Pediatrics and of Microbiology and Immunology, Stanford University School of Medicine

---

[1] The National Academies of Sciences, Engineering, and Medicine's planning committees are solely responsible for organizing the workshop, identifying topics, and choosing speakers. The responsibility for the published Proceedings of a Workshop rests with the workshop rapporteurs and the institution.

CHRISTIAN SINCLAIR, Outpatient Palliative Oncology Lead, Division of Palliative Medicine, University of Kansas Medical Center, representing the American Academy of Hospice and Palliative Medicine

Project Staff

LAURENE GRAIG, Director, Roundtable on Quality Care for People with Serious Illness
SYLARA MARIE CRUZ, Research Associate
RAJBIR KAUR, Senior Program Assistant
SHARYL NASS, Director, Board on Health Care Services, and Director, National Cancer Policy Forum
INDIA OLCHEFSKE, Research Associate (until June 2019)
ANDREW M. POPE, Director, Board on Health Sciences Policy

Consultant

JOE ALPER, Consulting Writer

ROUNDTABLE ON QUALITY CARE FOR PEOPLE WITH SERIOUS ILLNESS[1]

LEONARD D. SCHAEFFER (*Chair*), Judge Robert Maclay Widney Chair and Professor, University of Southern California

JAMES A. TULSKY (*Vice Chair*), Chair, Department of Psychosocial Oncology and Palliative Care, Dana-Farber Cancer Institute; Chief, Division of Palliative Medicine, Brigham and Women's Hospital; Professor of Medicine and Co-Director, Center for Palliative Care, Harvard Medical School

JENNIFER BALLENTINE, Executive Director, The California State University Institute for Palliative Care

ROBERT A. BERGAMINI, Medical Director, Palliative Care Services, Mercy Clinic Children's Cancer and Hematology, representing the Supportive Care Coalition

AMY J. BERMAN, Senior Program Officer, The John A. Hartford Foundation

LORI BISHOP, Vice President of Palliative and Advanced Care, National Hospice and Palliative Care Organization

PATRICIA A. BOMBA, Vice President and Medical Director, Geriatrics, Excellus BlueCross BlueShield

SUSAN BROWN, Senior Director, Health Education, Susan G. Komen

GRACE B. CAMPBELL, Assistant Professor, Department of Acute and Tertiary Care, University of Pittsburgh School of Nursing, representing the Association of Rehabilitation Nurses

STEVE CLAUSER, Director, Healthcare Delivery and Disparities Research Program, Patient-Centered Outcomes Research Institute

PATRICK CONWAY, President and Chief Executive Officer-Elect, Blue Cross and Blue Shield of North Carolina

DAVID J. DEBONO, Medical Director, Oncology, Anthem Inc.

CHRISTOPHER M. DEZII, Lead, Quality and Measure Development, State and Federal Payment Agencies, U.S. Value, Access and Payment, Bristol-Myers Squibb

---

[1] The National Academies of Sciences, Engineering, and Medicine's forums and roundtables do not issue, review, or approve individual documents. The responsibility for the published Proceedings of a Workshop rests with the workshop rapporteurs and the institution.

ANDREW DREYFUS, President and Chief Executive Officer, Blue Cross Blue Shield of Massachusetts
CAROLE REDDING FLAMM, Executive Medical Director, Blue Cross Blue Shield Association
MARK B. GANZ, President and Chief Executive Officer, Cambia Health Solutions
ZIAD R. HAYDAR, Senior Vice President and Chief Clinical Officer, Ascension Health
PAMELA S. HINDS, Director of Nursing Research and Quality Outcomes, Children's National Health System
HAIDEN HUSKAMP, 30th Anniversary Professor of Health Care Policy, Harvard Medical School
KIMBERLY JOHNSON, Associate Professor of Medicine, Senior Fellow in the Center for the Study of Aging and Human Development, Duke University School of Medicine
CHARLES N. KAHN III, President and Chief Executive Officer, Federation of American Hospitals
REBECCA A. KIRCH, Executive Vice President of Healthcare Quality and Value, National Patient Advocate Foundation
TOM KOUTSOUMPAS, Co-Founder, Coalition to Transform Advanced Care
SHARI M. LING, Deputy Chief Medical Officer, Center for Clinical Standards and Quality, Centers for Medicare & Medicaid Services
BERNARD LO, President and Chief Executive Officer, The Greenwall Foundation
JOANNE LYNN, Director, Center for Elder Care and Advanced Illness, Altarum Institute
DIANE E. MEIER, Director, Center to Advance Palliative Care
AMY MELNICK, Executive Director, National Coalition for Hospice and Palliative Care
JERI L. MILLER, Chief, Office of End-of-Life and Palliative Care Research, and Senior Policy Analyst, Division of Extramural Science Programs, National Institute of Nursing Research, National Institutes of Health
R. SEAN MORRISON, Director, National Palliative Care Research Center

BRENDA NEVIDJON, Chief Executive Officer, Oncology Nursing Society
HAROLD L. PAZ, Executive Vice President and Chief Medical Officer, Aetna Inc.
JUDITH R. PERES, Long Term and Palliative Care Consultant, Clinical Social Worker and Board Member, Social Work Hospice and Palliative Care Network
PHILLIP A. PIZZO, Founding Director, Stanford Distinguished Careers Institute, Former Dean and David and Susan Heckerman Professor of Pediatrics and of Microbiology and Immunology, Stanford University School of Medicine
THOMAS M. PRISELAC, President and Chief Executive Officer, Cedars-Sinai Health System
JOANNE REIFSNYDER, Executive Vice President, Clinical Operations and Chief Nursing Officer, Genesis Healthcare, representing the Hospice and Palliative Nurses Association
RACHEL ROILAND, Director, Serious Illness Care Initiative, National Quality Forum
JUDITH A. SALERNO, President, The New York Academy of Medicine
DIANE SCHWEITZER, Acting Chief Program Officer, Patient Care Program, Gordon and Betty Moore Foundation
KATRINA M. SCOTT, Oncology Chaplain, Massachusetts General Hospital, representing the Association of Professional Chaplains
KATHERINE SHARPE, Senior Vice President, Patient and Caregiver Support, American Cancer Society
JOSEPH W. SHEGA, Regional Medical Director, VITAS Hospice Care, representing the American Geriatrics Society
CHRISTIAN SINCLAIR, Outpatient Palliative Oncology Lead, Division of Palliative Medicine, University of Kansas Medical Center, representing the American Academy of Hospice and Palliative Medicine
SUSAN ELIZABETH WANG, Regional Lead for Shared Decision-Making and Advance Care Planning, Southern California Permanente Medical Group, Kaiser Permanente

Roundtable on Quality Care for People with Serious Illness Staff

LAURENE GRAIG, Director, Roundtable on Quality Care for People with Serious Illness
SYLARA MARIE CRUZ, Research Associate
RAJBIR KAUR, Senior Program Assistant
INDIA OLCHEFSKE, Research Associate (until June 2019)
MICAH WINOGRAD, Financial Officer
SHARYL NASS, Director, Board on Health Care Services, and Director, National Cancer Policy Forum
ANDREW M. POPE, Director, Board on Health Sciences Policy

Reviewers

This Proceedings of a Workshop was reviewed in draft form by individuals chosen for their diverse perspectives and technical expertise. The purpose of this independent review is to provide candid and critical comments that will assist the National Academies of Sciences, Engineering, and Medicine in making each published proceedings as sound as possible and to ensure that it meets the institutional standards for quality, objectivity, evidence, and responsiveness to the charge. The review comments and draft manuscript remain confidential to protect the integrity of the process.

We thank the following individuals for their review of this proceedings:

HAILEY W. BULLS, Moffitt Cancer Center
JESSICA MERLIN, University of Pittsburgh
BOB TWILLMAN, University of Kansas School of Medicine

Although the reviewers listed above provided many constructive comments and suggestions, they were not asked to endorse the content of the proceedings nor did they see the final draft before its release. The review of this proceedings was overseen by **SARA ROSENBAUM,** The George Washington University. She was responsible for making certain that an independent examination of this proceedings was carried out in accordance with standards of the National Academies and that all review comments were carefully considered. Responsibility for the final content rests entirely with the rapporteurs and the National Academies.

Acknowledgments

The National Academies of Sciences, Engineering, and Medicine's Roundtable on Quality Care for People with Serious Illness wishes to express its sincere gratitude to the Planning Committee Co-Chairs, Andrew Dreyfus and James Tulsky, for their valuable contributions to the development and orchestration of this workshop. The roundtable also wishes to thank all of the members of the planning committee, who collaborated to ensure a workshop complete with informative presentations and rich discussions. Finally, the roundtable thanks the speakers and moderators, who generously shared their expertise and their time with workshop participants.

Support from the many annual sponsors of the Roundtable on Quality Care for People with Serious Illness is critical to the roundtable's work. The sponsors include Aetna Inc., Altarum Institute, American Academy of Hospice and Palliative Medicine, American Cancer Society, American Geriatrics Society, Anthem Inc., Ascension Health, Association of Professional Chaplains, Association of Rehabilitation Nurses, Blue Cross Blue Shield Association, Blue Cross Blue Shield of Massachusetts, Blue Cross and Blue Shield of North Carolina, Bristol-Myers Squibb, The California State University Institute for Palliative Care, Cambia Health Solutions, Cedars-Sinai Health System, Center to Advance Palliative Care, Centers for Medicare & Medicaid Services, Coalition to Transform Advanced Care, Excellus BlueCross BlueShield, Federation of American Hospitals, The Greenwall Foundation, The John A. Hartford Foundation,

Hospice and Palliative Nurses Association, Kaiser Permanente, Susan G. Komen, Gordon and Betty Moore Foundation, National Coalition for Hospice and Palliative Care, National Hospice and Palliative Care Organization, National Palliative Care Research Center, National Patient Advocate Foundation, National Quality Forum, The New York Academy of Medicine, Oncology Nursing Society, Patient-Centered Outcomes Research Institute, Social Work Hospice and Palliative Care Network, Supportive Care Coalition, and the National Academy of Medicine. The roundtable is grateful to the MAYDAY Fund for its generous support for this workshop.

Contents

ACRONYMS AND ABBREVIATIONS   xix

PROCEEDINGS OF A WORKSHOP   1
INTRODUCTION   1
UNDERSTANDING THE OPIOID USE DISORDER EPIDEMIC AND ITS IMPACT ON PATIENTS, FAMILIES, AND COMMUNITIES   9
PAIN MANAGEMENT FOR PEOPLE WITH SERIOUS ILLNESS: CHALLENGES AND OPPORTUNITIES IN THE CONTEXT OF THE OPIOID USE DISORDER EPIDEMIC   17
    A Patient's Perspective on Opioid Use in Serious Illness, 18
    Opioid Correction Versus Opioid Trauma: Where Policy Meets Chronic Pain, 20
    Disparities in Access to Pain Medications, 25
    Pain Management for Children with Serious Illness: Challenges and Opportunities in the Context of the Opioid Use Disorder Epidemic, 30
    Discussion, 33
ADDRESSING THE CHALLENGE OF PATIENTS WITH COMORBID SUBSTANCE USE DISORDER AND SERIOUS ILLNESS   36
    Discussion, 42

IMPACT OF POLICY AND REGULATORY RESPONSE TO THE
OPIOID USE DISORDER EPIDEMIC ON THE CARE OF PEOPLE
WITH SERIOUS ILLNESS   44
    State Policies Addressing the Opioid Use Disorder Epidemic, 45
    A Federal Perspective on Policies and Regulatory Approaches, 49
    A Payer's Perspective on Policies to Address the Opioid Use
      Disorder Epidemic, 52
    Discussion, 53
CARING FOR PEOPLE WITH SERIOUS ILLNESS IN THE
CONTEXT OF THE OPIOID USE DISORDER EPIDEMIC:
LESSONS TO INFORM POLICY AND PRACTICE   56
    Discussion, 62
REFERENCES   69

APPENDIX A: Statement of Task   77
APPENDIX B: Workshop Agenda   79

Boxes, Figures, and Table

BOXES

1 Suggestions Made by Individual Workshop Participants to Improve Pain Management for People with Serious Illness in the Context of the Opioid Use Disorder Epidemic, 5
2 Summary of Key Themes Raised at the Workshop, 57

FIGURES

1 Increase in opioid prescribing, 10
2 Rates of opioid pain reliever (OPR) overdose deaths, OPR treatment admissions, and kilograms of OPR sold, 1999–2010, 11
3 Age-adjusted rates of death related to prescription opioids and heroin drug poisoning in the United States, 2000–2014, 14
4 Drugs involved in U.S. overdose deaths, 1999–2017, 15
5 U.S. mortality rates have risen because of the opioid use disorder epidemic, 15
6 Equality versus equity, 27
7 Perceptions of disparities in health care, 28
8 An algorithm for deciding what actions to take with patients with serious illness who display behaviors suggestive of a substance use disorder, 40
9 Drug poisoning mortality: United States, 2016, 46

xvii

TABLE

1 Definitions of Health Care Disparities, 26

Acronyms and Abbreviations

AMA	American Medical Association
CBD	cannabidiol
CDC	Centers for Disease Control and Prevention
CMS	Centers for Medicare & Medicaid Services
DEA	Drug Enforcement Administration
DSM-V	*Diagnostic and Statistical Manual of Mental Disorders, 5th Edition*
FDA	Food and Drug Administration
HHS	U.S. Department of Health and Human Services
IOM	Institute of Medicine
MAT	medication-assisted treatment
NGA	National Governors Association
NIH	National Institutes of Health
NOWS	neonatal withdrawal syndrome

OPR	opioid pain reliever
PDMP	prescription drug monitoring program
PQ-MSAS	PediQUEST Memorial Symptom Assessment Scale
SAMHSA	Substance Abuse and Mental Health Services Administration
STORM	Stratification Tool for Opioid Risk Management
VA	U.S. Department of Veterans Affairs

Proceedings of a Workshop

INTRODUCTION[1]

The United States is facing an opioid use disorder epidemic, with opioid overdoses killing more than 47,000 people in 2017 (NASEM, 2019). The past three decades have witnessed a significant increase in the prescribing of opioids for pain, based on the belief that patients were being undertreated for their pain coupled with a widespread misunderstanding of the addictive properties of opioids. This increase in prescribing of opioids also saw a parallel increase in addiction and overdose. The 2000s saw a wave of overdose deaths driven by the increased use of illegal drugs such as heroin. Currently, the nation is in the midst of another wave of overdose deaths due to the increased use of synthetic opioids such as fentanyl (CDC, 2018). In an effort to address this ongoing epidemic of opioid misuse, policy and regulatory changes have been enacted that have served to limit the availability of prescription opioids for pain management.

Overlooked amid the intense focus on efforts to end the opioid use disorder epidemic is the perspective of clinicians who are experiencing a

---

[1] The planning committee's role was limited to planning the workshop, and the Proceedings of a Workshop was prepared by the workshop rapporteurs as a factual summary of what occurred at the workshop. Statements, recommendations, and opinions expressed are those of individual presenters and participants, and are not necessarily endorsed or verified by the National Academies of Sciences, Engineering, and Medicine, and they should not be construed as reflecting any group consensus.

significant amount of daily tension as opioid regulations and restrictions have limited their ability to treat the pain of their patients facing serious illness. Increased public and clinician scrutiny of opioid use has resulted in patients with serious illness facing stigma and other challenges when filling prescriptions for their pain medications or obtaining the prescription in the first place. Thus, clinicians, patients, and their families are caught between the responses to the opioid use disorder epidemic and the need to manage pain related to serious illness.

The Roundtable on Quality Care for People with Serious Illness of the National Academies of Sciences, Engineering, and Medicine sponsored a workshop on November 29, 2018, to examine these unintended consequences of the responses to the opioid use disorder epidemic for patients, families, communities, and clinicians, and to consider potential policy opportunities to address them. The workshop, Pain Management for People with Serious Illness in the Context of the Opioid Use Disorder Epidemic, unfolded over five sessions.

- The opening session provided context with an overview of the scope and severity of the opioid use disorder epidemic.
- The second session focused on how responses to the epidemic affect the ability of people with serious illness to access opioid medications for pain. Workshop speakers shared clinicians' perspectives on their ability to effectively treat their patients' pain, discussed disparities in access to pain medications, and discussed issues related to pain management for seriously ill infants and children.
- Pain management needs of those with comorbid substance use disorder and serious illness were examined in the workshop's third session.
- The workshop's fourth session focused on policy and regulatory responses to the opioid use disorder epidemic, including federal and state regulatory policy, as well as payment policy. Speakers in the fourth session discussed measures that have been developed and implemented to address the opioid use disorder epidemic and whether those measures have been sufficiently flexible to limit unintended consequences for those with serious illness. Policies to expand access to non-opioids for pain management were also examined, as were associated coverage and reimbursement policies.
- The final session of the workshop aimed to identify actionable next steps by focusing on areas such as improving professional medical

education to better prepare clinicians to treat and manage pain and addiction, enhancing the development of, and access to, alternatives to opioids, and expanding access to treatment for substance use disorder.

The Roundtable on Quality Care for People with Serious Illness serves to convene stakeholders from government, academia, industry, professional associations, nonprofit advocacy groups, and philanthropies. Inspired by and expanding on the work of the Institute of Medicine (IOM)[2] report *Dying in America: Improving Quality and Honoring Individual Preferences Near the End of Life* (IOM, 2015), the roundtable aims to foster ongoing dialogue about crucial policy and research issues to accelerate and sustain progress in care for people of all ages experiencing serious illness.

In his introduction to the workshop, James Tulsky, chair of the Department of Psychosocial Oncology and Palliative Care at the Dana-Farber Cancer Institute, said that when he moved to Massachusetts in 2015, it became clear that clinicians and members of Dana-Farber's outpatient palliative care service were experiencing great angst over how to care for people suffering from pain related to their cancer in the context of the opioid use disorder epidemic. Massachusetts, he noted, has been hit particularly hard and was working to develop solutions to address the epidemic. In describing the increased difficulty clinicians faced in obtaining access to opioids for their patients as a result of heightened regulatory oversight of opioid prescribing, Tulsky observed: "They are trying to figure out a way to thread the needle."

Andrew Dreyfus, president and chief executive officer of Blue Cross Blue Shield of Massachusetts, explained in his introductory remarks that caring for people with serious illness and opioid use disorder is a major concern for his organization. He pointed out that in 2012, his organization was one of the first in the nation to begin to focus on changing the culture of opioid prescribing by implementing a "comprehensive" opioid utilization program on opioid prescribing rates, which included formal agreements between patient and provider, a requirement for the payer's approval prior to new opioid prescriptions and quantity limits.[3] Some of the policies his

---

[2] As of March 2016, the Health and Medicine Division of the National Academies of Sciences, Engineering, and Medicine continues the consensus studies and convening activities previously carried out by the Institute of Medicine (IOM). The IOM name is used to refer to publications issued prior to July 2015.

[3] For more information, see https://www.cdc.gov/mmwr/volumes/65/wr/mm6541a1.htm (accessed April 1, 2019).

organization developed have since been adopted by others and endorsed by the Centers for Disease Control and Prevention (CDC). At the same time, Blue Cross Blue Shield of Massachusetts began looking holistically and more broadly at issues that served as barriers to treating opioid use disorder, such as cost sharing and administrative constraints. In addition to its commitment to combatting the opioid use disorder epidemic, the organization made a public commitment to focus on improving care for people with serious illness including offering more end-of-life benefits.[4]

Dreyfus noted that both of these health issues share many similarities: Patients with chronic pain and those with substance use disorder have suffered from being outside of the mainstream of medical treatment. Both illnesses are highly influenced by the social circumstances of patients and their families' dynamics, as well as the emotional and behavioral health issues of patients and their families.

This Proceedings of a Workshop summarizes the presentations and discussions. The speakers, panelists, and workshop participants presented a broad range of views and ideas. Box 1 provides a summary of suggestions for potential actions from individual workshop participants. Appendix A contains the workshop's Statement of Task and Appendix B contains the workshop agenda. The workshop's speakers' presentations (as PDF and audio files) have been archived online.[5]

---

[4] For more information, see https://www.bostonglobe.com/business/2015/12/27/blue-cross-expands-benefits-for-end-life-care/5Uduttll3fG3ARVZkktP8I/story.html (accessed April 1, 2019).

[5] For more information, see http://nationalacademies.org/hmd/Activities/HealthServices/QualityCareforSeriousIllnessRoundtable/2018-NOV-29.aspx (accessed January 18, 2019).

BOX 1
Suggestions Made by Individual Workshop Participants to Improve Pain Management for People with Serious Illness in the Context of the Opioid Use Disorder Epidemic

Advancing Patient-Centered Care
- Accept that that there will be different solutions for each patient. (Humphreys)
- Allow for treatment to be decided by the patient and his or her physician. (Harris)
- Ensure that the Centers for Disease Control and Prevention (CDC) opioid prescribing guideline is used appropriately. (Botticelli, Friedrichsdorf, Kertesz, Meghani)
- Increase access to palliative care and pain specialists who are trained to screen for opioid use disorder and to treat opioid use disorder in the palliative care setting. (Smith)
- Treat patients through a constant risk–benefit analysis. (Merlin)

Improving the Treatment of Pain Among the Seriously Ill Pediatric Population
- Determine not whether it is appropriate to use opioids to treat pain in children, but rather, what amount of opioid prescribing is appropriate in children. (Friedrichsdorf)
- Expand access to interdisciplinary pediatric outpatient pain clinics, inpatient services, mental health services, and drug treatment programs covered by health insurance. (Friedrichsdorf)
- Separate the pediatric agenda to address the need to prescribe opioids for children with serious illness from the adult agenda. (Steinhorn)
- Create designated CDC pediatric guideline and have pediatric pain specialists on panels that develop guidelines given children ages 0–17 years represent 22 percent of the U.S. population. Currently all guidelines and recommendations including the guideline published by CDC are made for people older than 18. (Friedrichsdorf)

Focusing on Patient Outcomes
- Be concerned with patient outcomes instead of the number of pills prescribed. (Kertesz, Smith)

continued

BOX 1 Continued

- Collect and publicly report patient outcomes, including whether they are dead or alive, if their care has been continuous or if they have lost care, whether they were hospitalized or not, when collecting metrics on prescription numbers, and be held accountable for adverse outcomes. (Kertesz)
- Assess the current capacity of each state to deal with the epidemic and to identify evidence-based and promising practices that they can deploy and evaluate not just in terms of reducing the number of prescriptions filled or overdose deaths, but also in terms of patient outcomes. (Tewarson)

Addressing Stigma and Stereotypes
- Challenge assumptions about who has substance use disorder. (Harris)
- Address the societal stigma that patients with chronic pain are now sharing with those who have substance use disorders by educating the nation that chronic pain and substance use disorder are both health conditions. (Nickel)
- Change the current narrative that stereotypes people of color as the problem when, in fact, White suburban and rural populations have seen the greatest rise in opioid-related deaths. (Smith)
- Change the language surrounding substance use disorder to be neutral and judgment free. (Merlin)

Improving Provider Education and Support
- Respond to and support providers who have been traumatized by the harm they have caused their patients by restricting access to pain medications. (Kertesz)
- Reverse metrics, policies, and legal threats that jeopardize protection of legacy patients—patients who were on opioids prior to new regulations[a]—nearly all of which violate the CDC guideline while invoking their authority. (Kertesz)
- Improve the way clinicians are trained to treat pain. (Smith)
- Better educate physicians about how to manage pain with modalities other than opioids. (Alford)
- Train all providers to be competent in how to assess and manage pain, prescribe opioids safely, and assess and manage opioid use disorder. (Alford, Harris)
- Educate providers to do a better job of securing opioid medications and limit the number of short-term prescriptions they are writing. (Wargo)

- Alleviate the fear clinicians have today regarding prescribing opioids to those who would legitimately benefit from them by creating a safe harbor, which will require a robust statement from a public authority such as CDC, the American Medical Association (AMA), and perhaps the Drug Enforcement Administration (DEA), that clinicians will be protected in these situations. (Kertesz)
- Provide the clinicians with support, mentoring, and training in appropriate opioid prescribing. (Kertesz)
- Invest in multidisciplinary faculty development to meet the need for board-certified pain specialists and substance use disorder specialists. (Alford)
- Increase clinicians' understanding of the role that trauma, particularly adverse childhood events and exposure to intergenerational substance use disorder, plays in determining the risk of developing a substance use disorder. (Nickel)
- Increase communication between clinicians in the chronic pain and serious illness world and clinicians in the substance use disorders field. (Tulsky)

Enhancing Treatment and Prevention of Pain and Substance Use Disorder
- Acknowledge that pain and substance use disorder may occur together and treat both. (Merlin)
- Use comprehensive treatments for patients with pain and a substance use disorder that includes access to naltrexone. (Harris)
- Increase efforts to prevent substance use disorder by delaying the age of first use of drug, alcohol, and tobacco use by providing pediatricians and primary care physicians with the knowledge to teach parents and their adolescent patients how to protect themselves from this illness. (Nickel)
- Include early detection and intervention in efforts to solve the problem of substance use disorder. (Nickel)

Expanding Research and Knowledge Dissemination
- Conduct studies on the effects of mandated policies and collect data on adverse events, particularly suicidality. (Kertesz)
- Create a clearinghouse for all of the educational materials that organizations such as CDC, the Food and Drug Administration, AMA, the American College of Physicians, and many specialty societies have produced. (Alford)

continued

BOX 1 Continued

- Conduct more research on the intersections among serious illness, pain management, and substance use disorders. (Merlin)
- Include the technology industry in addressing the opioid use disorder epidemic. (Liebschutz)

Pursuing Policy and Regulatory Opportunities
- Change policy to allow methadone clinics, in particular, and substance use disorder treatments in general, to be incorporated into routine medical care and the medical health care system. (Humphreys, Merlin)
- Permanently change reimbursements under Medicare and Medicaid so that substance use disorder treatments are reimbursed at the same level as cancer and heart disease. (Humphreys)
- Expand medication-assisted treatment (MAT) for individuals with substance use disorder, with a focus on providing resources to community health centers across the nation as a means of increasing access to treatment in rural areas and creating better integration with primary care. (Botticelli)
- Revise the 50-year-old federal methadone regulations to allow for more integration into primary care. (Botticelli)
- Accelerate the collection, analysis, and dissemination of data to help policy makers. (Botticelli)
- Eliminate barriers to MAT, such as the need for prior approvals for those who have insurance, eliminating copays, and providing appropriate reimbursement for individuals covered by Medicare or Medicaid. (Harris)
- Ensure physicians are using their state's prescription drug monitoring program as a data tool. (Harris)
- Enforce legislation, which was passed by Congress but not acted on by the DEA, to allow for partial fills of opioid medications. (Alford, Twillman)
- Address the barriers to sharing data included in 42 CFR Part 2, which deals with the confidentiality of substance use disorder patient records. (Tewarson)

[a] For more information, see https://www.emsworld.com/news/12309641/-legacy-patients-pay-the-price-in-opioid-crackdowns (accessed March 6, 2019).

UNDERSTANDING THE OPIOID USE DISORDER EPIDEMIC AND ITS IMPACT ON PATIENTS, FAMILIES, AND COMMUNITIES

The workshop's first session began with a video featuring Laura Martin, substance use prevention coordinator for the city of Quincy, Massachusetts. Martin shared the story of how her younger brother became addicted to opioids and later died from a heroin overdose in his childhood bedroom just days after being released from a self-committed, 30-day treatment facility and shortly before starting law school. Martin noted how the stigma attached to opioid use disorder inhibits individuals with the disorder and their families from seeking help. This stigma, she stressed, has had the effect of limiting the resources the nation has put into providing evidence-based treatment and support for those who suffer from an opioid use disorder. She also spoke about the multigenerational effect the opioid use disorder epidemic is having on families, as grandparents and even great-grandparents are left to care for their grandchildren and great-grandchildren.

Following the video, Jane Liebschutz, professor of medicine and chief of the Division of General Internal Medicine at the University of Pittsburgh Medical Center, provided a historical perspective on opioid prescribing and substance use disorders. She also reviewed the criteria for a diagnosis of opioid use disorder; examined the impact of the opioid use disorder epidemic; and briefly discussed treatment options for the disorder.

Liebschutz traced the roots of the current epidemic to the discovery made 200 years ago, when German pharmacist Friedrich Wilhelm Adam Sertürner isolated the molecule, which he named morphine, from poppy seeds and determined that 15 milligrams of morphine should be the standard dose for anesthesia, but not oversedation, and this dose is still used today. Liebschutz explained that morphine was first used to treat pain among wounded soldiers during the Civil War—the first time morphine was used for a large patient population.

In 1899, said Liebschutz, Bayer introduced heroin—a chemical derivative of morphine—as a new medication for chronic cough; by 1914, the addictive properties of medicinal opioids were recognized. As a result, the U.S. Congress passed the Harrison Act of 1914 (approved on December 17, 1914, and effective on March 1, 1915) that regulated non-medical opioid use and made possession of an opioid illegal without a prescription.

Liebschutz explained that a half-century later, in the 1960s and 1970s, heroin use was largely a problem of minority communities, inner cities, and returning Vietnam veterans. In fact, to combat the high rates of opioid use disorder in Vietnam veterans, in 1972 the Nixon administration approved methadone as a treatment. At about the same time, there was a new sense within the medical community that patients with serious pain, particularly patients with cancer, were being undertreated with opioids. A 1973 study by Marks and Sachar found that despite being treated with narcotic analgesics for pain, 32 percent of medical inpatients continued to experience severe distress, and another 41 percent were in moderate distress. Liebschutz pointed out that in 1980, a letter was published in the *New England Journal of Medicine* claiming that those treated with narcotics rarely developed addiction. The letter suggested that those who were given opioids for pain would not develop addiction (Jick et al., 1970; Porter and Hick, 1980). "Many of us, including myself, really did think that for a long time," said Liebschutz.

Based on the belief that patients in serious pain were undertreated and that opioids were not addictive, opioid prescribing soared in the early 1990s (see Figure 1). In 1996, Purdue Pharma developed OxyContin, a long-acting form of oxycodone, and marketed it as a painkiller with a lower potential for addiction. In 2001, the Joint Commission determined that

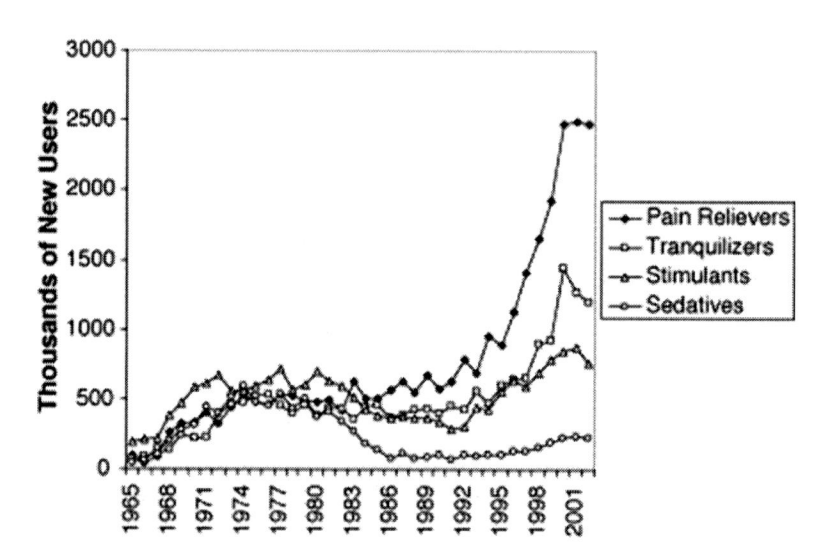

FIGURE 1 Increase in opioid prescribing.
SOURCES: As presented by Jane Liebschutz, November 29, 2018; Compton and Volkow, 2006.

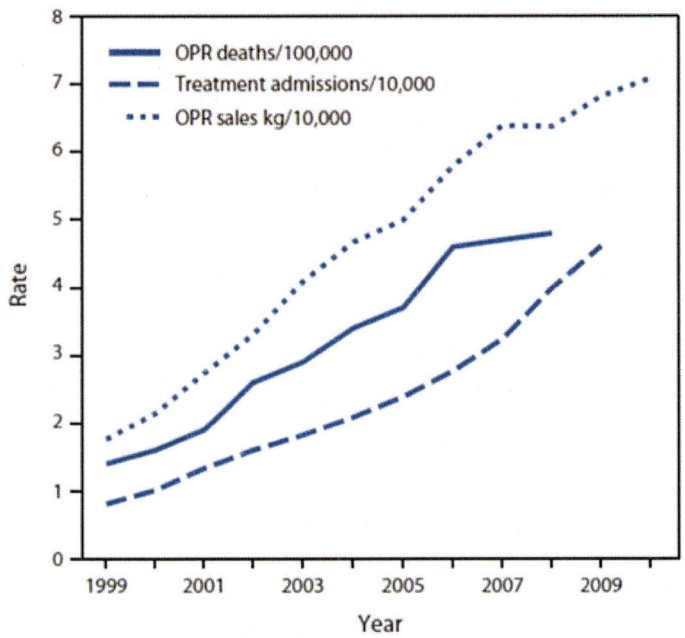

FIGURE 2 Rates of opioid pain reliever (OPR) overdose deaths, OPR treatment admissions, and kilograms of OPR sold, 1999–2010.
SOURCES: As presented by Jane Liebschutz, November 29, 2018; Paulozzi et al., 2011.

pain should be the fifth vital sign,[6] and that hospitals and health care programs would be graded on how well they were treating their patients' pain. However, "the parallel rise in opioid prescription also went along with the parallel increase in addiction and overdose," Liebschutz explained (Paulozzi et al., 2011) (see Figure 2).

Liebschutz pointed out that addiction is a brain disease in which drugs "hijack" the brain's natural dopamine-powered reward circuits (Volkow et al., 2016). According to Liebschutz, normally, these circuits become active when someone engages in joyful activities. Early in the use of addictive drugs, a person feels euphoric, and withdrawal produces a mild reduction in energy. A user looks forward with excitement to using the drug again. With time and further use, neuroadaptation,[7] a learning process in which the

---

[6] The other vital signs are blood pressure, pulse rate, rate of respiration, and temperature.
[7] For more information, see https://www.ncbi.nlm.nih.gov/pmc/articles/PMC3870778 (accessed April 1, 2019) and https://www.ncbi.nlm.nih.gov/pmc/articles/PMC2886284 (accessed April 1, 2019).

brain reacts to a previously inexistent sensory input and its ability to adapt to it by ignoring it or using it properly (Alió and Pikkel, 2014), occurs. This process reduces the euphoria to merely feeling good when using the drug, and the mild reduction in energy due to withdrawal becomes reduced energy. Instead of looking forward to using, the individual starts to "really desire" the drug. As the neuroadaptation continues, the drug does not make the individual feel good, but merely helps them escape dysphoria, a state of unease or dissatisfaction with life. Depression, anxiety, and restlessness affect the individual when the drug is not present, and as a result, the individual starts obsessing over obtaining the drug. At the same time, a cognitive learning process occurs along with this neuroadaptation (Lewis, 2018).

Liebschutz reviewed the diagnostic criteria for opioid use disorder, as listed in the fifth edition of the *Diagnostic and Statistical Manual of Mental Disorders, 5th Edition* (DSM-V) (APA, 2013). Symptoms include

- Use in larger amounts or over a longer period than intended;
- Unsuccessful efforts to cut down/persistent use;
- A great deal of time spent getting, using, or recovering from use;
- Craving, or a strong desire to use;
- Recurrent use resulting in failure to fulfill major obligations at work, school, or home;
- Continued use despite social or interpersonal problems caused by use;
- Social, work, and/or recreational activities given up or reduced;
- Use in situations in which it is physically hazardous;
- Continued use despite physical or psychological harm;
- Withdrawal; and
- Tolerance.

Liebschutz particularly emphasized the last two criteria—tolerance and withdrawal—and noted that patients who take opioids as prescribed can have these particular symptoms of opioid use disorder without having the disorder. For example, patients with end-stage cancer can develop withdrawal and tolerance, but that does not mean they have a substance use disorder. Similarly, a baby whose mother had the disorder can exhibit withdrawal and tolerance, but does not have a substance use disorder. Patients must exhibit more symptoms that these two to be diagnosed with substance use disorder, explained Liebschutz.

Noting that the terms "substance abuse" and "opioid abuse" are no longer used, Liebschutz explained that the correct terminology is "mild, moderate, or severe opioid use disorder," depending on whether the patient displays two to three, four to five, or six or more of the above symptoms in 12 months, respectively.

Tracing the early period of the opioid use disorder epidemic, Liebschutz described the emergence of so-called "pill mills." These are pharmacies affiliated with a physician who, for cash, would administer a minimal examination and prescribe an outsized number of pills, explained Liebschutz. She observed that those pharmacies were responsible for a significant amount of "opioids being diverted and also [for] feeding addiction that had developed during this period of time." She explained that states responded by creating prescription drug monitoring programs (PDMPs), which are state-based databases used to identify patients who "doctor shop" for multiple opioid prescriptions and clinicians who overprescribe. By 2018, all but one state had created such databases—the Missouri legislature has blocked the creation of a database there.[8] Liebschutz explained that law enforcement has used these databases to aggressively pursue overprescribers and shutter nearly all pill mills.

Liebschutz pointed out that while such overprescribing and relatively easy access to opioid painkillers created the first wave of the opioid use disorder epidemic, the second wave (see Figure 3) arose when Mexican drug cartels realized they could produce heroin and market it directly to suburban and rural White customers, bypassing the inner cities. She noted that in 2010, there was an inflection point in the number of heroin deaths while prescription opioid deaths started to level off. Liebschutz stated that this is not necessarily a one-to-one substitution of people switching from prescription opioids to heroin, but instead is an indication of "heroin in and of itself being a problem" said Liebschutz. Liebschutz further pointed out that in 2002, an estimated 400,000 Americans had used heroin in the previous year, but by 2016, the number had risen to nearly 1 million.

Liebschutz explained that the third wave of the opioid use disorder epidemic is currently sweeping the United States, driven by fentanyl, a synthetic opioid that is 50 times more potent than heroin and 100 times more potent than morphine. Largely manufactured in China, fentanyl is smuggled into the country in small quantities, making it difficult for law enforcement to interdict. Liebschutz explained that drug dealers mix fentanyl with heroin to increase the intensity of the high. Carfentanil, an

---

[8] The workshop was held in November 2018; the Missouri House voted to approve a statewide PDMP on February 11, 2019 (Dabbs, 2019).

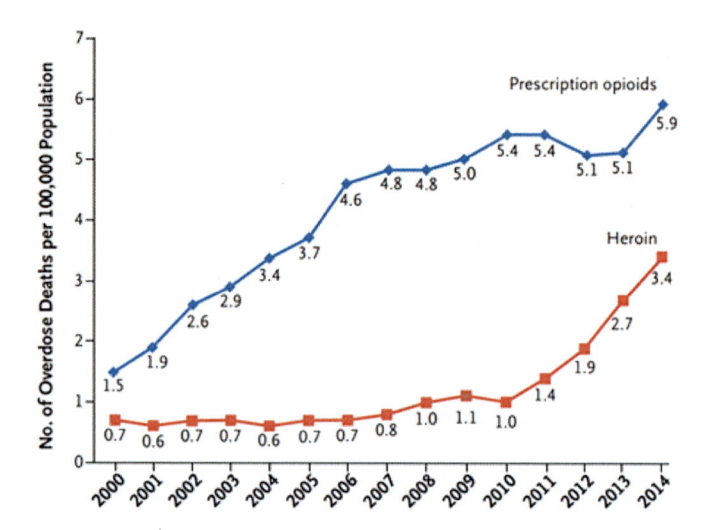

FIGURE 3 Age-adjusted rates of death related to prescription opioids and heroin drug poisoning in the United States, 2000–2014.
SOURCES: As presented by Jane Liebschutz, November 29, 2018; Compton et al., 2016.

elephant tranquilizer 10,000 times more potent than morphine, has been implicated in a number of deaths around the country, she added.

Drug overdoses killed more than 72,000 Americans in 2017 (see Figure 4), with the biggest increase over the past few years caused by fentanyl overdose. Liebschutz explained that because of fentanyl's potency, people experimenting without knowing exactly what they are getting from their dealers have suffered unintentional overdoses that now dwarf all other causes. Perhaps the most astonishing outcome from the dramatic rise in overdose deaths is that the U.S. mortality curve is bending upward for U.S. non-Hispanic, middle-aged Whites (see Figure 5) for the first time in more than four decades (Case and Deaton, 2015). Notably, the mortality rate of U.S. Hispanics follows the trends of other countries. According to Case and Deaton, this rise in mortality among U.S. non-Hispanic Whites is due to what is referred to as the "deaths of despair": overdose, alcoholism, and suicide (Case and Deaton, 2015).

As Liebschutz alluded to at the start of her presentation, the opioid use disorder epidemic is having a significant impact on families. In 2010, 5.4 million lived in a household headed by grandparents, up from 4.7 million in 2005 (Scommegna, 2012). The number of grandparents raising grand-

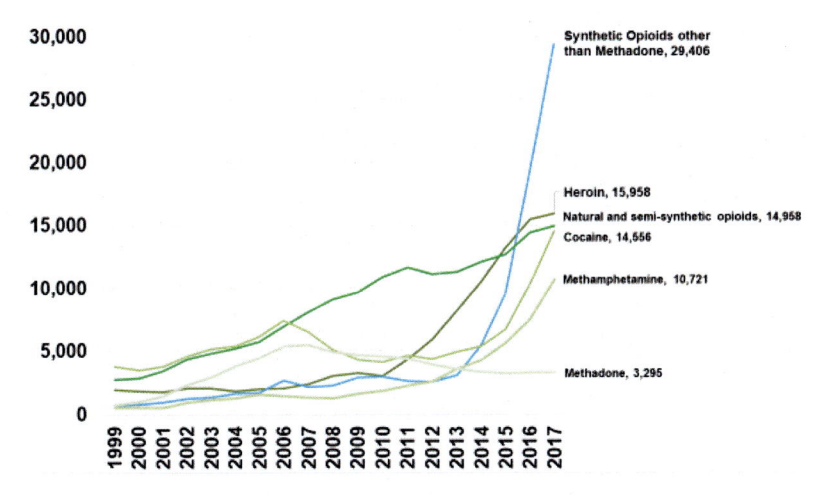

FIGURE 4 Drugs involved in U.S. overdose deaths, 1999–2017.
SOURCE: As presented by Jane Liebschutz, November 29, 2018.

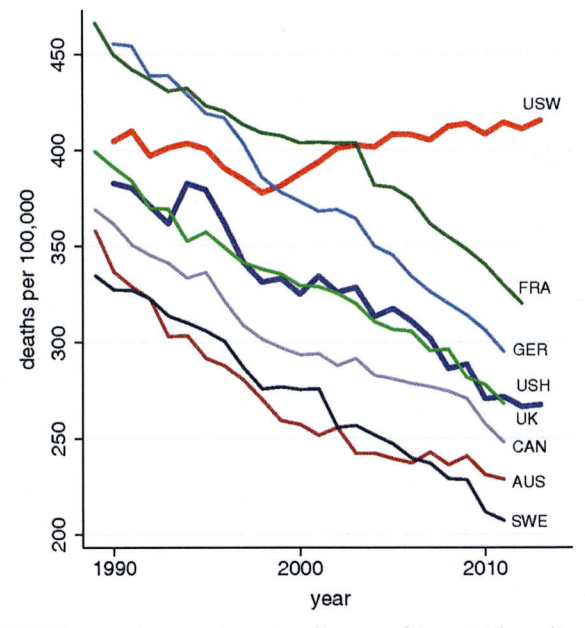

FIGURE 5 U.S. mortality rates have risen because of the opioid use disorder epidemic.
NOTE: AUS = Australia; CAN = Canada; FRA = France; GER = Germany; SWE = Sweden; UK = United Kingdom; USH = U.S. Hispanics; USW = U.S. White non-Hispanics.
SOURCES: As presented by Jane Liebschutz, November 29, 2018; Case and Deaton, 2015.

children increased by 7 percent from 2009 to 2016, with 2.7 million grandparents raising grandchildren (Cancino, 2016). Liebschutz noted there are a number of support groups for parents affected by the opioid use disorder epidemic, including Learn to Cope[9] and Parents of Addicted Loved Ones.[10]

Liebschutz pointed out that neonatal abstinence syndrome, now called neonatal withdrawal syndrome (NOWS), has risen in the United States from 1.19 per 1,000 live births in 2009 to 5.63 per 1,000 live births (Stover and Davis, 2015). NOWS is characterized by hyperactivity of the central and autonomic nervous system and the gastrointestinal tract. Babies affected by NOWS do not meet the criteria of addiction according to the DSM-V (as described earlier) but are born with physical dependence. Not all babies of mothers who use opioids develop NOWS. The incidence of NOWS is higher in rural areas than in urban areas. As of 2015, in West Virginia—an epicenter of the opioid use disorder epidemic—some 50 babies out of 1,000 are born with this condition (Umer et al., 2018).

Turning to the issue of medications for opioid use disorder, Liebschutz pointed out that the three types of approved medications include full agonists (methadone and off-label morphine in the United States) that activate the opioid receptors, resulting in full opioid effect; partial agonists (buprenorphine, also called Suboxone) that activate the receptors to a lesser degree; and antagonists (naltrexone, also called Vivitrol) that block opioids by attaching to the receptors without activating them (NAABT, 2016). Naloxone, brand name Narcan, is a different type of medication that does not treat opioid use disorder but instead is a reversal agent used to treat overdoses.

Methadone is only dispensed by federally licensed facilities, usually in locations removed from populated areas, and requires dosing that is observed daily, although some patients receive take-home methadone after long periods of sobriety. A 30-day supply of buprenorphine can be given in any outpatient setting, and the Drug Enforcement Administration (DEA) will issue a waiver after special training. Naltrexone can be given by any licensed prescriber without a waiver through an oral form daily or an injectable form every 4 weeks.

A meta-analysis of all-cause mortality during and after either methadone or buprenorphine treatment found that all-cause mortality for methadone treatment was 11.3 per 1,000 versus 36.1 per 1,000 for individuals off treatment. For buprenorphine, the comparable figures were

---

[9] For more information, see http://www.learn2cope.org (accessed January 25, 2019).
[10] For more information, see http://palgroup.org (accessed January 25, 2019).

4.3 per 1,000 for those on treatment versus 9.5 per 1,000 for those who are out of treatment (Sordo et al., 2017). Liebschutz added that observational data from Massachusetts have shown that future mortality of individuals who have experienced a non-fatal overdose and are prescribed either methadone or buprenorphine is about one-third of those who are not on treatment (Larochelle et al., 2018). "These are life-saving medicines," said Liebschutz.

Behavioral therapies studied as adjuvants to medication include cognitive-based therapies and contingency management. The bottom line after hundreds of studies, said Liebschutz, is that adding behavioral therapy to medication therapy appears to provide no extra benefit to patients. "This is not to say that people will not benefit in some ways from therapy, but it doesn't necessarily result in improvement in substance use outcomes," she said. She believes most treatment programs still require adjunctive behavioral therapy because it is a vestige of years of treatment practice.

In summary, Liebschutz said that since the discovery of opioid medications, balancing therapeutic use with the potential for addiction has been critical. The brain, she noted, has a strong adaptive mechanism to opioids, which influences many of the subsequent harms and behaviors. The urgency of this issue is clear given that the opioid use disorder epidemic is bending the mortality curve in the United States and negatively affecting a growing number of children and families. Liebschutz concluded that fortunately, medications to treat opioid use disorder exist, and those treatments do save lives.

PAIN MANAGEMENT FOR PEOPLE WITH SERIOUS ILLNESS: CHALLENGES AND OPPORTUNITIES IN THE CONTEXT OF THE OPIOID USE DISORDER EPIDEMIC

Building on Liebschutz's introductory presentation, R. Sean Morrison, the Ellen and Howard C. Katz Professor and chair of the Brookdale Department of Geriatrics and Palliative Medicine at the Icahn School of Medicine at Mount Sinai, started the second session by highlighting one of the key themes of the workshop. He pointed out that although it has always been assumed that laws and regulations are not meant to limit the use of opioids for people who are dying or have cancer, there are millions of Americans with serious illness who do not have cancer, who are not dying, and yet who are living in pain and genuinely benefit from the analgesic effects of opioids. For those individuals, said Morrison, the lack of access and ability to obtain these medications can have real consequences. He emphasized that research clearly shows that pain is undertreated in this country and that untreated pain has real consequences, including chronic pain syndromes, disability, and a negative impact on quality of life.

A Patient's Perspective on Opioid Use in Serious Illness

To provide real-world context for how opioids serve as life-saving medications for someone with a serious illness who suffers from chronic pain, Morrison introduced Rosanne Leipzig, the Gerald and May Ellen Ritter Professor in the Brookdale Department of Geriatrics and Palliative Medicine at the Icahn School of Medicine at Mount Sinai, and her wife Ora Chaikin, who for the past 25 years has suffered from a painful condition that destroys her tendons and joints. More than a decade ago, Leipzig asked Morrison if he would serve as the palliative care physician for Chaikin, and he has cared for her since that time.

Leipzig explained that she approached Morrison after consulting with multiple clinicians who were not only unable to provide a diagnosis for Chaikin's condition, but could not successfully address the extreme pain she was experiencing. When Chaikin first saw Morrison, the pain in her hands and feet made it difficult to walk or perform activities of daily living. Over the subsequent few years, the pain increased and spread to other joints, including her shoulders and back. Her feet and hands, meanwhile, were deforming because her tendons were "breaking," according to Chaikin; she has endured multiple surgeries to replace her shoulders and reconstruct her feet.

Chaikin said her relationship with opioids has been difficult. "When I initially started the opioids, I would periodically flush them down the toilet or throw them in the trash because I did not want to be taking them, and I did not want to be labeled an addict or become dependent," she said. "I felt I could beat this some other way." Eventually, she accepted that opioids had to be part of her life if she was ever going to be able to function at a high level. Not long afterward, she received a letter from her pharmacy benefit company informing her that it was cutting in half the amount of opioids she could receive. Reversing that decision, she said, took many weeks, during which time she went into withdrawal. Even today, she worries that at any moment her access will be restricted once again, and she has been told by various people that she has to get off opioids. "I am made to feel really like an addict," said Chaikin.

In fact, when a new owner took over the pharmacy that Chaikin had used for 30 years, he told her that he did not want people like her in his store and that he would lose his license if he filled her prescription. In a store filled with people, the new owner screamed at Chaikin, calling her an addict. According to Chaikin, the worst part of taking opioids is the judgment from others.

Chaikin explained that when using a mail order pharmacy, her prescriptions are only filled if she submits extra paperwork. The resulting delays in receiving her medication lead her to start tapering her dosage so that she will not run out of medication, but the result is that her pain increases. With regard to functioning and her quality of life, "these medications have made all the difference in the world," Leipzig observed.

Morrison noted that Chaikin has tried multiple non-opioid therapies over the years and has rotated which opioids she takes to minimize various side effects. At one point, Morrison prescribed an extended-release formulation of hydromorphone, which allowed Chaikin to go through the day without taking a pill every 3 hours. However, that drug has been pulled from the market.

Leipzig recounted one incident when Chaikin received letters from their insurance company informing her that it was reducing the amount of medication she could receive. Morrison, Chaikin's treating physician, was not notified of this change, and all the pharmacists could do was say they were sorry, telling her "rules are rules." This problem was not resolved until Leipzig happened to be serving on a panel with the insurance company's chief medical officer and she explained the situation to him directly. Six weeks later, the issue was resolved.

In closing, Morrison noted that Chaikin is not an exception. "I have an entire panel of people like Ora," he said. "They are quiet, and they feel this is only them, that they are not empowered, and they feel pretty powerless and helpless." Leipzig added that she is tired of hearing that there is no evidence that opioids work for chronic pain, stating that a lack of evidence is not the same as having evidence of no effect. "I do not know how we get people to recognize this, but there is an N of one right here," said Leipzig, pointing to her wife. "Somehow, we need to get the word out."

With Chaikin and Leipzig providing a compelling real-life perspective of the challenges of treating patients with serious illness and chronic pain, Morrison then introduced the three panelists who would further address the issue: Stefan Kertesz, professor in the Division of Preventive Medicine at the University of Alabama at Birmingham School of Medicine; Cardinale Smith, associate professor of medicine and director of quality for cancer services at the Mount Sinai Health System and the Brookdale Department of Geriatrics and Palliative Medicine at the Icahn School of Medicine at Mount Sinai; and Stefan Friedrichsdorf, medical director in the Department of Pain Medicine, Palliative Care, and Integrative Medicine at the Children's Hospitals and Clinics of Minnesota. An open discussion followed the three panelists' presentations.

Opioid Correction Versus Opioid Trauma: Where Policy Meets Chronic Pain

"This is a time of tragedy, and times of tragedy call for questions," said Kertesz, referring to the rising number of opioid overdose deaths in the United States. The questions he raised include

- How do we know what we think is right is actually right?
- Could what seems right be wrong?
- For whom might it not be right?

Kertesz pointed out that from the mid-1990s until 2012, opioids were vastly overprescribed, which caused harm warranting a systems-level decline in opioid prescribing (Kertesz and Gordon, 2018). Forced reductions in opioid prescribing, however, are now highly incentivized or even mandated for those patients who have been on opioids over the long term. He argued that this violates both the ethical and evidentiary norms traditionally applied to medical practice. "The adverse consequences of this are evident, and better approaches are available to us," Kertesz emphasized.

Kertesz recounted a case of a 73-year-old veteran who had painful polyarthritis and had received a renal transplant in 2003. He had been prescribed opioids since 2001 at doses ranging from an equivalent of 105 to 140 milligrams of morphine, but for reasons not documented in his electronic health record, his dose was reduced by several 30 to 60 percent cuts between 2014 and 2016, to the equivalent of 22.5 milligrams of morphine by 2017. Kertesz said the patient accepted all of this without protest, but he suffered a progressive loss of energy and the ability to organize himself and keep track of his medications. In March 2017, this patient was admitted to Kertesz's inpatient hospital service with progressive failure of his transplanted kidney. "The acute rejection would have been prevented had he been able to keep up with his medicines that were intended to prevent a rejection of the transplanted kidney," said Kertesz. Unfortunately, a mixture of pain and passivity led the patient to lose his ability to do so.

After dialysis stabilized the patient, Kertesz increased his opioid dose modestly and notified his physician that he had probably gone too far in reducing the dosage. However, within 3 weeks of his release from the hospital, the patient's dose was cut in half, and he was readmitted twice in the next 6 months. The patient passed away shortly after that time.

For Kertesz, this case raises two policy questions. First, was this person's opioid reduction considered favorable according to metrics used by the National Committee for Quality Assurance, the Centers for Medicare & Medicaid Services (CMS), the Office of the Inspector General at the U.S. Department of Health and Human Services (HHS), the U.S. Department of Veterans Affairs (VA), the U.S. Department of Justice, and by all potential payers? If the answer, he said, is yes, then the second question this case raises is whether the tapering of his dosage protected the patient from harm. Because the patient died, Kertesz explained, the answer is probably no. "That really gets to the heart of the matter," he said. "Where the metrics in play to reverse a very large and very serious crisis are neutral on the question of whether patients live or die."

Kertesz noted that his patient had not gone through acute withdrawal, but rather experienced what is called prolonged abstinence syndrome. In fact, this patient never qualified for a diagnosis of opioid use disorder as described in DSM-V. Some patients, he said, do feel better and have more energy after a slow opioid taper. Others, however, go through sedating medications, adopt other ineffective procedures, suffer medical deterioration and loss of care relationships, turn to other illicit substances or alcohol, or become suicidal. By his count, some 50 suicides have been reported publicly in the news or social media that mention both pain and opioid reduction; he emphasized that this does not determine a cause-and-effect relationship. He has reviewed two of these cases in depth and they are quite complicated, he added.

As an aside, Kertesz explained that injectable opioids, such as fentanyl, injectable morphine, and injectable Dilaudid, have been in short supply over the past 2 years, which has affected inpatient treatment of acute pain. In April 2018, the American Society of Health–System Pharmacists reported that 86 percent of medical facilities indicated that shortages were having a moderate to severe effect. They identified the consequences of such shortages as swapping products and formulations (ASHP, 2018); daily deliberations among pharmacists, nurses, and doctors that led to medical errors in some cases; and limiting the responsibility of opioid care to a small group of specialized providers (Bruera, 2018). These shortages are largely the result of manufacturing shortfalls, with some contribution from today's tightly regulated supply chain, he added.

The CDC guideline for prescribing opioids for chronic pain calls on physicians to back away from the tendency to prescribe opioids on the premise that they are not routinely superior to other treatments for chronic pain.[11] The CDC guideline also calls for evaluating the risks and benefits of prescribing opioids because these drugs are deeply problematic due to their highly addictive nature and recommend clinicians prescribe the lowest effective dose. For patients already taking opioids, the guideline calls on clinicians to evaluate the harm versus the benefits for that individual patient, though they do not provide a dose target and do not mandate dose reductions (Dowell et al., 2016). Kertesz noted that although the guideline does represent a reasonable consensus of experts, the evidence supporting this guideline was generally of low quality.

Overall, the nation's response to the opioid use disorder epidemic has been to control prescriptions by tightening product supply and imposing quality indicators based on pill dose and count, noted Kertesz. In addition, 28 states have passed laws regulating opioid dosage (NCSL, 2018). Payers, in essence, are imposing non-consensual tapering, pharmacies are invoking their own liability and responsibilities to reject prescriptions, and physicians are operating under fear of investigation. As a result, said Kertesz, "a single prescription is now subject to multiple, high-stakes, and often conflicting imperatives."

Kertesz then provided some examples of how these conflicting mandates are playing out in practice. One example he shared was a 2018 form letter sent from a medical practice to its patients, which stated that CMS had implemented a new law mandating that opioid doses not exceed a maximum of 90 equivalents of morphine. The law this letter cited, however, was a state law. Kertesz noted that incorrect legal citations by authorities are commonly used to taper patients off opioids. Some institutions are sending letters to patients informing them they will be tapered by more than 10 percent per week, stating that most patients have less pain with lower doses, which Kertesz said reflects inferences not supported by the evidence. In some cases, institutions are offering group support, cannabidiol (CBD), or buprenorphine as replacements for opioids.

---

[11] For more information on the CDC Guideline for Prescribing Opioids for Chronic Pain, see https://www.cdc.gov/drugoverdose/prescribing/guideline.html (accessed April 1, 2019).

Kertesz also cited a letter from a chain pharmacy to a provider prescribing opioids stating that the pharmacy would no longer fill that provider's prescriptions for controlled substances without including the specific metric used to justify this action. "This is a letter that effectively blackballs the doctor and their patients forever from that pharmacy if controlled substances are involved," said Kertesz, who added that many of these letters were issued around the time that many chain pharmacies were named as defendants in combined multidistrict litigation. Additionally, he pointed out that both-Individual pharmacies are also restricting access. In one instance, a patient received a letter requiring medical records, including imaging results and doctors' notes, and a recent urine drug test that was positive for the opioid, before the pharmacy would fill the patient's prescription. According to Kertesz, this is little more than a liability reduction exercise that "positions the pharmacist as the assessor of pain care quality." Additionally, he pointed out that both insurance coverage policies and state Medicaid programs can mandate dose reductions that the CDC guideline did not endorse.[12]

Kertesz noted that federal prosecutors also are becoming involved. In 2018, for example, the U.S. Attorney's Office in Atlanta identified 30 top prescribers of opioids in the Atlanta area, even though the U.S. Department of Justice noted it had not determined if those 30 physicians had broken any laws. Kertesz said such efforts are part of the U.S. Department of Justice's initiative to reduce opioid prescriptions by one-third over the next 3 years. "Will the threat of prison reduce prescribing?" he asked. In his view, he said it probably would.

Kertesz also noted that some health care organizations are highlighting their success in reducing opioid use, yet there is no discussion of how those reductions are affecting patient outcomes. Nationally, high-dose opioid prescribing fell 48 percent over 8 years, yet "the overdose deaths involving potentially prescribed opioids (i.e., natural and semisynthetic, excluding methadone, fentanyl, or heroin) remain constant at approximately 10,000 per year since 2010, according to a query from the U.S. National Vital Statistics System," according to a study by Kertesz and Gordon (2018). "To me, this signals we may not be pushing on the right string to get the result we want," Kertesz said.

The policy conundrum, said Kertesz, is that agencies have prioritized opioid counts as the indicator of quality, safety, and good faith, and most invoke the CDC guideline inaccurately. Opioid counts have become the

---

[12] This text has been revised since prepublication release.

de facto standards for legal risk and professional liability, which makes any patient who receives any longstanding prescription for opioids, but especially at high doses, a liability to all concerned. "What do professionals normally do with liabilities?" asked Kertesz. They "get rid of them," he answered. He noted there is a case to be made that tapering, whether consensual or not, is helpful to some individuals, but the science on institutionally mandated tapering requires additional discussion. The bottom line, in his view, is that policy has moved ahead of the science, with the crucial missing piece being that the agencies mandating these policies do not measure, nor are they accountable for, patient outcomes, including mortality associated with these policies.

There is, however, another layer to the response to the opioid use disorder epidemic, and that has to do with how health systems respond to and support their clinicians who have been traumatized by the harm they have caused their patients by restricting their access to pain medications. In health care, said Kertesz, the normal response to a catastrophic event is root cause analysis, remediation, investigation, and the offer of support. For deaths related to opioids stoppage or taper, those customary responses to patient harms are conspicuously lacking. "This is a real departure from the normal way we practice health care," he said.

Regarding the data to support the new regulatory mandates, Kertesz noted that the literature suggests that many patients who voluntarily taper their use of opioids achieve good results (Frank et al., 2017). What is needed, Kertesz asserted, are studies on the effects of mandated policies and data on adverse events, particularly suicidality. For persons with diagnosable opioid use disorder involving prescription opioids, provision of buprenorphine-naloxone for a limited number of weeks followed by taper of that medication resulted in a failure rate of 91.4 percent (Weiss et al., 2011). Kertesz underscored that not all patients receiving long-term opioids would have qualified for this trial, but asserted that such poor results raise questions about tapering as a general policy for patients who have received opioids for pain on a long-term basis. One study also found high rates of suicidal ideation and suicidal self-direct violence in patients undergoing taper after long-term opioid use (Demidenko et al., 2017).

A better approach, said Kertesz, is to focus on the individual patients and the care they require, and not to treat all high-dose opioid users in the same way. He noted that high-dose opioid patients can have a compendium of serious medical, psychological, and substance use disorder-related morbidities that correlate highly with the receipt of high-dose opioids. "We can care for these conditions, and they are predictive of the very adverse outcomes that we want to prevent, which are overdose and suicide," said Kertesz. To make corrections at the systems level, he emphasized two key issues:

- A crucial step is to reverse metrics, policies, and legal threats that jeopardize protection of legacy patients; nearly all of these factors violate the CDC guideline while invoking its authority.
- Any entity using metrics based on prescription numbers must collect and publicly report patient outcomes, including whether they are dead or alive, if their care has been continuous or if they have lost care, and whether they were hospitalized or not, and be held accountable for adverse outcomes.

In closing, Kertesz pointed out that enacting health policy with no measurement of patient outcomes and no accountability is how the nation has gotten into the current mess. "This is a time of tragedy and a time for choosing," he said. "We professionals are implicated in creating this tragedy, and regulators are as well. We are under the gun, but so are our patients." While nobody at present has complete knowledge of what is right, he added, it is still important to ask how we know what we think is right is actually right.

Disparities in Access to Pain Medications

People of color overall disproportionately have higher morbidity and mortality rates when facing serious illness "and pain is a significant contributor to that," noted Cardinale Smith, who has personal experience with these challenges. Smith's 52-year-old father was diagnosed with Stage IV rectal cancer, and his physician at Mount Sinai prescribed a fentanyl patch to help relieve his pain. Smith, who was a fellow in oncology and palliative medicine at the time, went to five pharmacies in Brooklyn, where her father lived, before finally finding a pharmacy in Manhattan that could fill the prescription. Eventually, her father's physician changed dosing from every 72 hours to every 48 hours because that worked better for her father. The pharmacist accused Smith's father of diverting the patches, and called the prescribing physician and told him that fentanyl could not be dosed every 48 hours. As Smith remarked, the fact that she, as a clinician, could not get her father the care he needed underscores the problem facing those individuals who are not well versed in opioid prescribing, who are not health literate, and who cannot advocate for themselves.

Smith said there are several definitions of health care disparities put forth by different organizations (see Table 1). The definition she favors, from the National Institute on Minority Health and Health Disparities, notes that a certain population is a health disparity population if there is a significant difference in the overall rate of disease incidence, prevalence, morbidity, mortality, or survival rates in the population as compared to the health status of the general population. Smith also explained the difference between equality, which provides everybody with the same thing, and equity, which provides extra resources to those most in need (see Figure 6). Given the changing demographics of the nation, with minority populations, and particularly the Hispanic or Latino population, growing at a faster rate than the population as a whole, it is likely that there will be an increase in disparities when it comes to having access to pain medication, said Smith.

TABLE 1 Definitions of Health Care Disparities

Organization/ Group	Definition
CDC/Healthy People 2020	Type of difference in health that is closely linked with social or economic disadvantage. Health disparities negatively affect groups of people who have systematically experienced greater social or economic obstacles to health. These obstacles stem from characteristics historically linked to discrimination or exclusion such as race or ethnicity, religion, socioeconomic status, gender, mental health, sexual orientation, or geographic location.
IOM	Racial or ethnic differences in the quality of health care that are not due to clinical needs, preferences, and appropriateness of intervention.
NIH	Health disparities are differences in the incidence, prevalence, mortality, and burden of diseases and other adverse health conditions that exist among specific population groups in the United States.
NIMHD	A population is a health disparity population if there is a significant disparity in the overall rate of disease incidence, prevalence, morbidity, mortality, or survival rates in the population as compared to the health status of the general population.

NOTE: CDC = Centers for Disease Control and Prevention; IOM = Institute of Medicine; NIH = National Institutes of Health; NIMHD = National Institute on Minority Health and Health Disparities.
SOURCE: As presented by Cardinale Smith, November 29, 2018.

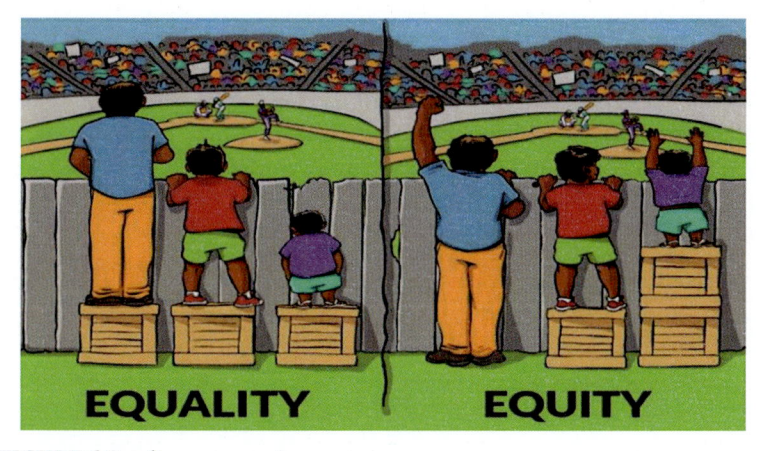

FIGURE 6 Equality versus equity.
SOURCES: As presented by Cardinale Smith, November 29, 2018; Interaction Institute for Social Change, Artist: Angus Maguire, interactioninstitute.org, madewithangus.com.

Chronic pain, said Smith, affects more people in the United States than common diseases such as cardiovascular disease, diabetes, and cancer, and there is an unequal burden of pain across racial and ethnic populations. In general, said Smith, different races and ethnicities self-report about the same rates of illicit drug use, but the rate of drug-induced deaths is far higher in whites than in Hispanics or African Americans.

The bottom line, said Smith, is that minority patients with pain have less access to pain medications and to the specialists who can prescribe them. They are also less likely to have their pain recorded, assessed, and treated, and are at increased risk for under-treatment of their pain. As Morrison noted earlier, there are real consequences of pain in terms of a person's ability to work and earn a living, with a significant impact on family dynamics.

There are many factors responsible for these disparities, said Smith, including health system–level factors such as PDMPs and the reluctance of pharmacies to fill prescriptions for opioids when the patient is a member of a minority population. At the clinician level, many providers lack knowledge about how to treat pain, operate on false stereotypes, and have implicit bias regarding minority populations and opioid use disorder. Patient-level factors include a fear of addiction and dependence that may be more prevalent in minority populations, as well as disparities in communication between patient and provider that arise during the clinical encounter.

Smith noted that a meta-analysis of multiple pain studies conducted between 1989 and 2011 found a significant gap in the quality of pain management that African Americans and Hispanics/Latinos received compared with Whites (Meghani et al., 2012). She added that another finding from this study was that Hispanics/Latinos and African Americans were more likely to receive non-opioid analgesics such as non-steroidal anti-inflammatory drugs. Similarly, a study looking at children up to age 21 who came to the emergency department with appendicitis found that African Americans were less likely to have their pain treated with opioids or any pain medication than were White children (Goyal et al., 2015).

Smith wonders how well-meaning, highly educated health care professionals working in their usual environment with a diverse population of patients can create a pattern of care that appears to be discriminatory. She does not believe her clinician colleagues are purposefully racist or discriminatory, but rather are discriminating because of imposed limitations and implicit bias. She noted studies from the Kaiser Family Foundation that sometimes asked physicians and always asked members of the public questions about how often they think health care systems treat people unfairly based on several criteria (Kaiser Family Foundation, 1999, 2002) (see Figure 7). The overall finding was that physicians believed disparities in care occurred less frequently than did the general public.

Generally speaking, how often do you think our health care system treats people unfairly based on…

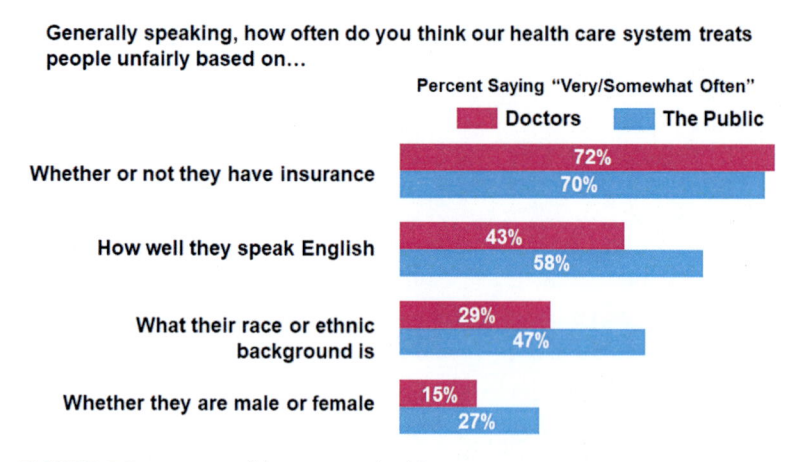

Percent Saying "Very/Somewhat Often" — Doctors / The Public

Criterion	Doctors	The Public
Whether or not they have insurance	72%	70%
How well they speak English	43%	58%
What their race or ethnic background is	29%	47%
Whether they are male or female	15%	27%

FIGURE 7 Perceptions of disparities in health care.
SOURCES: As presented by Cardinale Smith, November 29, 2018; Kaiser Family Foundation, 2002.

Another issue, noted Smith, is that physicians underestimate pain, particularly compared with how their patients perceive it. One study, for example, examined patients' and physicians' perceptions of chronic, non-cancer pain at 12 academic medical centers and found that "physicians are twice as likely to underestimate pain in Black patients compared to all other ethnicities combined" (Staton et al., 2007). However, researchers have found that even for patients who have been properly assessed and given a prescription of an opioid to treat their pain, those living in neighborhoods where the population was predominantly African American, Hispanic, or Asian had access to far fewer pharmacies with adequate opioid supplies compared with neighborhoods that were predominantly White (Morrison et al., 2000). One study in Michigan, which examined socioeconomic status and race, found that pharmacies in zip codes that contained large minority populations were less likely to carry "sufficient opioid analgesics" than those in zip codes with majority White populations regardless of income (Green et al., 2005).

Regarding PDMPs, Smith said there have been some studies on the impact of those programs on opioid prescribing rates, but few have looked at the effect of those programs on patient outcomes. "I would argue it is great to see numbers go down, but it is really the patient in front of us that matters," said Smith. One 2017 study found that the number of opioid prescriptions received by Medicaid recipients fell the most in states that have mandated that providers both register to be tracked in a drug monitoring system and use the system when making prescribing decisions for patients (Wen et al., 2017).

State laws are also contributing to limits on opioid prescriptions, said Smith. In New York, for example, the law requires a new prescription for someone with acute pain to be limited to 7 days of medication.[13] The law does exempt those with serious illness such as cancer or those in palliative care and hospice. Smith, who treats cancer patients, said that even when she writes a prescription in her health system's electronic health record and adds the correct diagnostic code, she still receives a call from the pharmacist making sure that she is prescribing the correct amount. "So, when you think about the barriers and the challenges that are put in place for clinicians who already are underestimating pain and not treating it as frequently in minority populations, one can imagine that that disparity only has the potential to increase," said Smith.

---

[13] For more information, see https://www.health.ny.gov/health_care/medicaid/program/update/2016/2016-07.htm#opioid (accessed March 6, 2019).

Smith also noted that health plans and pharmacies are developing their own rules and regulations about what they will or will not prescribe. Although she applauds those efforts, Smith said they have the effect of taking a medical decision out of the hands of the frontline clinicians. Her concern is that doing so could make it even more difficult for vulnerable populations to access and receive the treatment they need. "In trying to do well, we are creating an even bigger gap," said Smith. "We want to be able to provide the care that is best, but at the same time, limit the challenges that we are seeing."

In closing, Smith suggested that solutions to these challenges might start with changing the narrative from one that stereotypes people of color as the problem, given that the biggest rise in opioid-related deaths has been among White suburban and rural populations. In addition, said Smith, improvements must be made in the way clinicians are trained to treat pain, and access needs to increase to palliative care and pain specialists who are trained to screen for and treat opioid use disorder.

Pain Management for Children with Serious Illness: Challenges and Opportunities in the Context of the Opioid Use Disorder Epidemic

Shifting the focus to the pediatric perspective, Stefan Friedrichsdorf of the Children's Hospitals and Clinics of Minnesota opened his remarks by observing that, despite the fact that children ages 17 and younger make up more than 22 percent of the U.S. population (U.S. Census Bureau, 2014), the CDC guideline referred to by previous workshop speakers includes nothing about children—the guideline pertains to individuals age 18 years and older. Friedrichsdorf noted that no pediatricians were included in the working group that produced the guideline. Pain, according to Friedrichsdorf, is common, underrecognized, and undertreated in children (Friedrichsdorf et al., 2015). In fact, despite an increase in adult misuse of opioids, adults receive more pain medication than children with the same underlying condition (Beyer et al., 1983; Eland and Anderson, 1977; Schechter et al., 1986). In addition, said Friedrichsdorf, the younger the child is, the less likely they are to receive the appropriate analgesia to treat their pain (Broome et al., 1996; Ellis et al., 2002; Nikanne et al., 1999).

The problem with undertreating pain in children, explained Friedrichsdorf, is that children with persistent pain become adults with chronic pain, anxiety, and depression (Friedrichsdorf et al., 2016). In addition, inadequate analgesia for an initial procedure in children diminishes the effect of adequate analgesia in subsequent procedures (Weisman et al., 1998), while morbidity and mortality increases in preterm neonates who are undertreated for pain (Anand et al., 1999). Friedrichsdorf noted, too, that children with injury or acute burns are less likely to develop posttraumatic stress disorder in the months following treatment with higher doses of morphine (Nixon et al., 2010; Saxe et al., 2001; Stoddard et al., 2009).

By conservative estimates, there are 237,000 children ages 17 and under in the United States who are living with a life-limiting condition (Friedrichsdorf, 2017). In 1997, deaths attributed to all complex chronic conditions accounted for 7,242 infant deaths, 2,835 childhood deaths, and 5,109 adolescent deaths (Feudtner et al., 2001). On average, said Friedrichsdorf, children with advanced cancer at the end of life had a median of five symptoms, three causing high distress.[14] Friedrichsdorf identified three of these symptoms (dyspnea, cough, and pain) that would benefit from opioid treatment. Opioids, he said, are associated with many side effects and are potentially lethal, but "no other analgesics equal in potency and effect have been discovered or developed to reduce suffering" (Krane et al., 2018).

The opioid use disorder epidemic in the United States has produced "many experts, pundits, and politicians who really offer simplistic blameworthy origins for the problem," and "simplistic soundbites and solutions," said Friedrichsdorf. His views are shared by Krane and colleagues in a 2018 article. He noted that although physicians may be blamed for prescribing an opioid that leads to addiction and death of a previously healthy child, the fact is that the "first exposure to non-medical use of opioids in adolescents occurs most often from access to family members' or friends' prescriptions, not their own" (Krane et al., 2018). In a comprehensive article, Miech and colleagues concluded that "legitimate use of prescription opioids before high school completion does not predict opioid misuse after high school" (Miech et al., 2015).

On average, said Friedrichsdorf, people who die from a drug overdose have six medications in their bloodstream. Although dentists who prescribe too many opioid pills for a wisdom tooth extraction or root canal procedure need to be targeted, for example, the main problem with substance use disorders is that they are embedded in a "complicated matrix in our country of despair and hopelessness," said Friedrichsdorf. He noted that

---

[14] The median PediQUEST Memorial Symptom Assessment Scale (PQ-MSAS) total score was 9.3 in a study (Wolfe et al., 2015).

such despair and hopelessness correlates closely with socioeconomic factors such as unemployment, poor education, availability of illicit street opioids and diverted prescription opioids, a genetic predisposition to substance use disorder, and psychiatric conditions. There is scant evidence, he asserted, to support the existence of an epidemic of deaths resulting from the appropriate use of prescribed opioids (Krane et al., 2018). "How many children have to suffer needlessly from pain to avoid one opioid death?" asked Friedrichsdorf.

To counter the notion that prescribing morphine to a child with cancer will make it more likely that that child will be addicted to drugs when he or she grows up, Friedrichsdorf cited a study of more than 4,000 high school students. The study showed that medical use of prescription opioids without any history of non-medical use of prescription opioids is not associated with substance use behaviors at age 35 (McCabe et al., 2016). In contrast, adolescents who reported any history of non-medical use of prescription opioids did have an increased risk of substance use behaviors during adolescence (McCabe et al., 2007).

Friedrichsdorf also cited a study of public school students in Detroit. The study revealed that 76 percent of the students who were misusing an opioid by taking more than prescribed did so for pain relief only, while the other 24 percent of students did so to address non–pain relief motives (including experimentation, getting high, counteracting the effects of other drugs, safer than street drugs, and other motives). The study indicated that four out of five students in grades 7 to 11 who were prescribed opioids took them as prescribed (McCabe et al., 2013). Friedrichsdorf added that U.S. government statistics show that misuse of opioids among U.S. 12th graders has dropped dramatically despite the high overdose rates among adults (NIDA, 2017).

Many of the regulations applied to children and adolescents have no basis in scientific fact, noted Friedrichsdorf. For example, the Food and Drug Administration (FDA) has warned against prescribing tramadol to children because three children died over the past 50 years. Friedrichsdorf stressed that the question to ask is not whether it is appropriate to use opioids to treat pain in children, but rather, what amount of opioid prescribing is appropriate in children.

Friedrichsdorf and his colleagues take a multimodal approach to analgesia in children and use several different medications that act synergistically to provide more effective pediatric pain control with fewer side effects than would be achieved with a single analgesic. For acute pain, opioids are an important part of this approach in addition to adjuvant analgesia or to basic analgesia, according to Friedrichsdorf.

Friedrichsdorf pointed out that for chronic pain in children, opioids are actually contraindicated, and instead, he and his colleagues rely on physical and occupational therapy, integrative therapies, cognitive behavioral therapy, and getting children back into normal life. The problem, said Friedrichsdorf, is that few children in pain have access to clinics that offer these approaches to pain control, given that there are only eight functioning pediatric pain clinics in the nation. Even if a person happens to live near one of these clinics, insurers often refuse coverage for these evidence-based treatments. His clinic has a waiting list of 5,000 children. In fact, most children's hospitals do not have a designated inpatient pain team, and most insurers base reimbursements on adult guidelines that are not applicable to children.

In conclusion, Friedrichsdorf said that children in severe, acute pain are suffering today because adult experts crafted adult guidelines with no consideration of the 22 percent of the U.S. population that is under age 18. For Friedrichsdorf, withholding evidence-based analgesia to children is not only unethical, but also causes both immediate and long-term harm. While there are potential safety risks, such risks are manageable and do not justify denying administration of opioids to pediatric patients who have severe tissue injuries or who are at the end of their lives because of serious illness. In addition, he said, limiting access to pain clinics and appropriate pain medication risks driving adolescents in particular to illicit drugs that carry a much greater risk to their health and lives. Pediatric patients, he said, need access to interdisciplinary outpatient pediatric pain clinics, inpatient pediatric services, mental health services, and drug treatment programs covered by health insurance.

Discussion

During the discussion session following the speakers' presentations, workshop participant Diana Martins-Welch from Northwell Health asked the panelists if they had recommendations on how to treat patients with serious pain from Stage IV cancers and a history of substance use disorder. Although Kertesz pointed out that this topic would be covered in the next workshop session, he did note that his approach is to treat each individual differently, based on his or her unique situation. Some patients, for example, might need an extremely close monitoring program that involves knowledgeable nurses, while others might benefit from a non-opioid treatment.

Whatever the decision, he negotiates it up front through an explicit conversation with the patient.

Tulsky asked the panelists if the current attention paid to opioid use disorder reflects a racial bias, given that it has only come to prominence now that it is affecting White, rural communities. Smith replied that when illicit opioids were affecting minority communities, the response was that this was a legal justice system crisis, not a public health crisis, and the response was to put people in jail rather than treat their substance use disorder. She said "this only leads to and increases the bias."

Workshop participant Jack Rossfeld, a physician from Ohio, asked Kertesz if there are any policy demonstrations that measure patient outcomes, rather than pill counts. Kertesz replied that there are measurement tools to help determine who is at higher risk of developing an adverse outcome. The question then becomes what to do when such a tool identifies someone who is at high risk for an adverse outcome with opioids. He noted that the VA Stratification Tool for Opioid Risk Management (STORM) uses a real-time data dashboard to present an individual patient's risk level as well as patient-specific clinical risk factors (Oliva et al., 2017). What is missing, though, is evidence supporting what to do for those individuals who are at risk of adverse outcomes with opioids, most of whom have untreated mental health issues. There is no large trial proving how to get patients safely into care, according to Kertesz. He stressed the need for mentorship and support for primary care providers who prescribe opioids.

Workshop participant Marian Grant, a policy consultant and palliative care nurse practitioner, noted that she has seen the pendulum swing to where clinicians are now reluctant to prescribe opioids for patients with appropriate need. Recently, she explained, she had two cancer patients who used heroin, and one went back to using street drugs. The other patient, who was highly adherent with her methadone program, was struggling to deal with her pain without turning to street drugs. Grant's question to the panelists was what can be done to change the attitudes of clinicians, many of whom seem to have a "just say no" attitude to prescribing opioids. Kertesz said those clinicians need a safe harbor, which will require a robust statement from a public authority such as CDC, the American Medical Association (AMA), and perhaps the DEA, that they will be protected in these situations. His institution offers a consultative service where senior physicians can offer advice and support for difficult cases, but there is only so much safe harbor a senior doctor can provide. "We need insurers and officials to speak up," said Kertesz. Grant added that she was encouraged by a recent resolution[15] from AMA that pushed back at regulations that limit how doctors practice medicine.

As a palliative care clinician, Smith said she is comfortable managing pain and prescribing high doses of opioids when needed. However, what she has not learned is how to treat substance and opioid use disorder other than through an 8-hour course. Therefore, she is not comfortable treating substance and opioid use disorder. "I am fortunate that I have friends who are experts, but that is not true for the vast majority of clinicians who practice in this country," said Smith. Though her institution does have a substance use disorder clinic, she is unable to enroll her Medicaid patients in it.

Noting that he has heard from hospice medical directors that physicians in hospice settings refuse to write prescriptions for opioids and instead want the medical director to take the responsibility and possible liability of writing the opioid prescription, workshop participant Paul Tatum asked how to convince primary care providers that they are the best prescribers. Kertesz responded that, in fact, primary care providers might not be the best prescribers given that they may lack training on addiction, dependency, and treating pain. That said, it would not be practical to send every patient in need of an opioid prescription to the medical director of a hospice or palliative care program. "We are going to have to offer a degree of support and training that is beyond merely alluding to a guideline or a website," said Kertesz. In his opinion, those clinicians are clearly afraid and there is a need to address their fears with education, mentoring, and help.

Salimah Meghani from the University of Pennsylvania noted that the CDC guideline is of low quality, yet has been widely adopted by states, payers, insurers, pharmacists, and others as being evidence based. In her opinion, CDC and other federal agencies have turned a blind eye to the misapplication of the guideline (Meghani, 2016); this is particularly so in the case of pediatrics. At the same time, the President's Opioid Commission's report, issued in November 2017, recommends removing pain assessment from patient satisfaction surveys. Liebschutz questioned what could be done to increase the federal government's accountability regarding the widespread adoption of the CDC guideline. Friedrichsdorf said he did not have a good answer other than reworking the guideline with input from pediatricians and including evidence to support the guideline.

---

[15] For more information, see https://www.medpagetoday.com/meetingcoverage/ama/76322 (accessed April 1, 2019).

ADDRESSING THE CHALLENGE OF PATIENTS WITH COMORBID SUBSTANCE USE DISORDER AND SERIOUS ILLNESS

Jessica Merlin, associate professor of medicine in the Division of General Internal Medicine at the University of Pittsburgh, introduced herself as a general internist who trained in infectious diseases and palliative care and now practices as an addiction physician and behavioral scientist who runs a chronic pain clinic for people living with HIV/AIDS. She then provided some definitions for chronic pain, addiction or substance use disorder, and serious illness.

Chronic pain, explained Merlin, is distinguished from acute pain by duration, with chronic pain lasting at least 3 months (Interagency Pain Research Coordinating Committee, 2016; IOM, 2011). Chronic pain, she said, affects some 10 percent of the U.S. population (IOM, 2011). Although chronic pain can originate from an initial tissue injury, in some conditions, such as fibromyalgia or chronic lower back pain, the brain receives a strong pain signal even when there is no inflammation in the periphery. Chronic pain is not a symptom, observed Merlin, but is a chronic disease in and of itself. Thus, chronic pain is heavily influenced by biological, psychological, and social factors, and the optimal treatment should be multidisciplinary and include both pharmacological and non-pharmacological approaches.

Addiction, now called "substance use disorder," is also a chronic disease, Merlin explained, that hijacks the brain's pleasure reward system and can result in compulsive use of any number of substances, often simultaneously. As Liebschutz noted in her presentation, the DSM-V criteria for a substance use disorder includes a long list of items. Treatment involves both medication and psychosocial therapies.

Serious illness, said Merlin, is defined as a health condition that carries a high risk of mortality and either negatively affects a person's daily function or quality of life or excessively strains their caregivers (Kelley and Bollens-Lund, 2018). Examples of serious illness include cancer, pulmonary disease, congestive heart failure, renal failure, and dementia, among others.

Chronic pain, serious illness, and substance use disorder can intersect in a given patient in many ways, said Merlin (Paice, 2018). Chronic pain and substance use disorder are both common, and individuals who develop serious illness may already experience chronic pain, have a substance use disorder, or both. She noted that while pain and substance use disorder do not always occur together, addiction is more common in people with pain than in the general population. This may be because the opioids used to treat pain can be powerful triggers for addiction in people who are predisposed to it, or who have had a substance use disorder prior to developing chronic pain. In addition, pain is a common complication of serious illness, particularly as people live longer with their serious illness as a result of the development of new therapies. Moreover, serious illness can trigger a great deal of stress, which itself can exacerbate pain and be a powerful trigger for addiction. The result can be that individuals with serious illness will have chronic pain and develop a substance use disorder, Merlin explained.

Merlin said there is limited research at the intersection of serious illness, chronic pain, and substance use disorder despite it being an important clinical problem. In particular, there have been few studies on approaches for managing patients with serious illness, chronic pain, and a substance use disorder. The current literature focuses on patients with cancer in oncology and those in palliative care settings. Most cancer treatment programs, she said, do not screen their patients for opioid use disorder or substance use disorder risk (Tan et al., 2015). Those that do screen find that 20 to 40 percent of their patients have an elevated risk of opioid misuse when prescribed opioids for pain (Koyyalagunta et al., 2013; Ma et al., 2014; Yennurajalingam et al., 2018), and 10 percent report elevated and unhealthy alcohol use (Giusti et al., 2019). One study revealed that approximately 6 percent of cancer patients studied were diagnosed with a substance use disorder (Ho and Rosenheck, 2018). Merlin pointed out that concerning urine drug testing findings include toxicology results that are positive for substances not prescribed (e.g., cocaine, opioids that are not prescribed) or negative for substances that are prescribed (e.g., opioids). According to at least two studies, a significant share of oncology patients has these unexpected findings. In one study by Rauenzahn and colleagues, 46 percent of oncology patients at high risk for substance misuse tested positive for non-prescribed opioids, benzodiazepines, or potent illicit drugs such as heroin or cocaine. Thirty-nine percent of patients tested inappropriately negative (Rauenzahn et al., 2017). In another study, 54 percent of advanced cancer patients who were receiving chronic opioid therapy had abnormal urine drug test results (Arthur et al., 2016).

Merlin noted that pain management is an important component of palliative care, which is specialized medical care for people living with serious illness. It focuses on providing relief from the symptoms and the stress of serious illness to improve the quality of life for both the patient and family. She pointed out those individuals who have both pain and a substance use disorder often present to palliative care settings. Merlin and her colleagues conducted a national study of palliative care providers in which they asked about cancer survivors with chronic pain who were not at the end of life. More than half of the physicians and nurse practitioners who responded to the survey reported that they spend more than 30 minutes per day managing opioid misuse behaviors. At the same time, the respondents said that on a scale of 0 to 10, they rated their confidence in their ability to manage substance use disorder at a 5. Only 27 percent of the respondents reported having training or access to systems in place to address substance use disorder in their practices. Only 13 percent had a DEA waiver to prescribe buprenorphine, and 36 percent had no access to a substance use disorder specialist (Merlin et al., 2019).

Given the limited evidence base and the prevalence of comorbid serious illness, pain, and substance use disorder, Merlin and her colleagues have called for more research on:

- how to assess opioid risks, harms, and benefits in those with serious illness;
- what other pharmacological and non-pharmacological approaches might benefit patients;
- how to manage concerning behaviors tied to substance use disorder in patients with serious illness; and
- efforts in education and policy around these issues (Schenker et al., 2018).

In an effort to address the question of what clinicians should do when they have a patient with serious illness, pain, and a substance use disorder, Merlin looked to see whether the general literature on chronic pain and substance use disorder might inform possible approaches. Perhaps the first avenue to explore, she said, is to determine the optimal treatment for chronic pain in individuals with serious illness—regardless of whether they have a substance use disorder. Although the treatment of chronic pain and opioids are often conflated, the literature supports a multidisciplinary approach that can include opioids and other drugs, as well as non-pharmacologic therapies. Merlin emphasized that it is important to decide who should receive opioids and who should not, and to consider the risks versus the benefits of opioid therapy for each individual patient.

Merlin then raised the issue of whether there is a real distinction between "legitimate" or "organic" pain—pain that has an identifiable causes, such bone metastases, degenerative disc disease, or inflammatory conditions—and other types of pain such as idiopathic pain disorders. The message from the pain literature is clear that this distinction is not meaningful because chronic pain is not a symptom, but a disease in itself, regardless of the initial source of pain, explained Merlin. As a result, the idea that "organic pain" automatically merits treatment with opioids no longer holds true. "One needs to assess the risk versus benefits of prescribing opioids and not conflate opioids with good quality pain management," said Merlin.

Merlin spoke of the phenomenon known as pseudo-addiction, which is when someone continues to report pain and exhibits behaviors that may resemble a substance use disorder, when in fact they are not taking enough pain medication. These behaviors disappear when the amount of pain medication is increased. The pain and substance use disorder literature, Merlin said, clearly shows that pain and substance use disorder frequently coexist and that pseudo-addiction is a less than useful concept because there is little evidence to support it.

Merlin, along with Liebschutz and other colleagues, conducted a study in which they asked experts how they manage concerning behaviors that arise among patients on long-term opioid therapy. Such behaviors include missing appointments, taking opioids for symptoms other than pain, using more opioid medication than prescribed, asking for an increase in opioid dose, aggressive behavior, alcohol use, and use of other substances such as stimulants, heroin, and cannabis, in primary care settings (Merlin et al., 2018). From this study, the researchers came to a consensus on a complicated algorithm that would lead to recommended actions (see Figure 8). This approach starts with determining a diagnosis of the questionable behavior and reeducating the patient about the importance of taking opioids safely and not using illicit substances. It involves trying to understand if a pattern indicative of a substance use disorder is present, and if so, to treat that substance use disorder using evidence-based therapies.

Merlin noted that diagnosing a substance use disorder is challenging in individuals on long-term opioid therapy using the DSM-V criteria. This is due to the fact that those criteria were developed for people who are using opioids from non-medical sources.

One of the key issues is the stigma associated with long-term opioid use and substance use disorder, Merlin said. Referring to substance use disorder as a brain disease can help frame it in a way that is far less stigmatizing. Doing so is important, said Merlin, because patient outcomes are worse when providers use stigmatizing language. "This is not about political correctness," said Merlin. "This has real implications." Instead of the

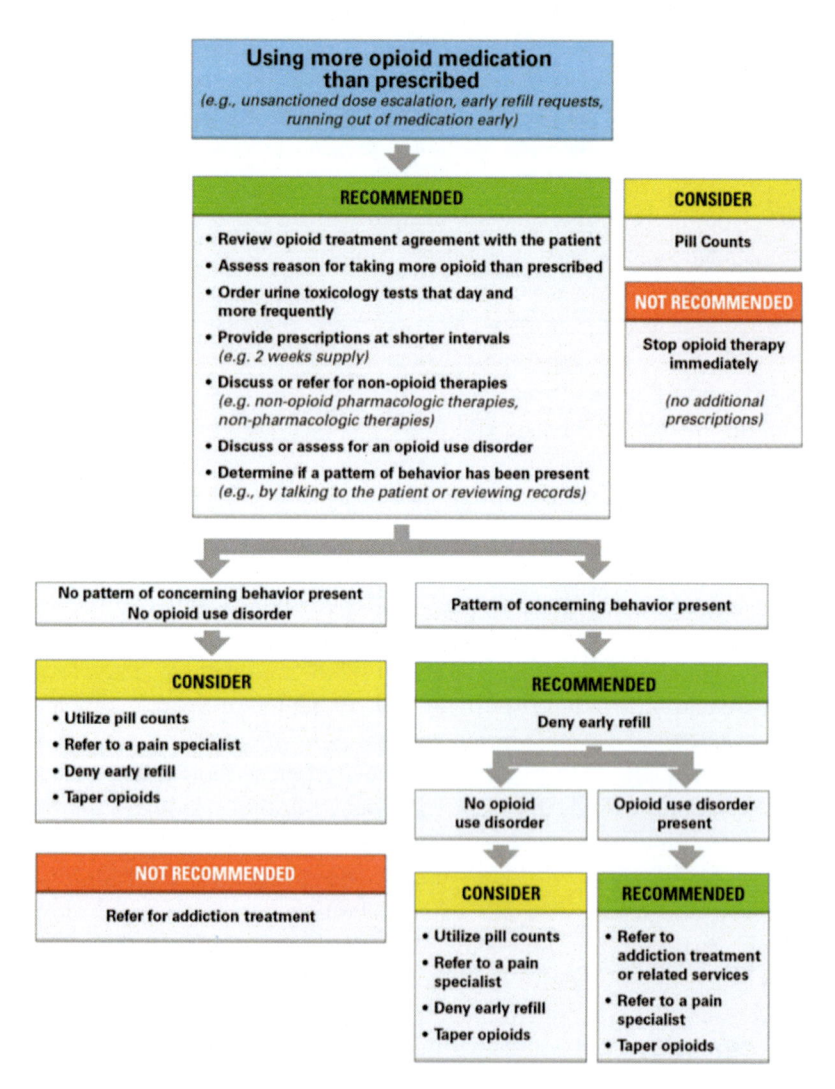

FIGURE 8 An algorithm for deciding what actions to take with patients with serious illness who display behaviors suggestive of a substance use disorder.
NOTE: For additional information, see http://mytopcare.org/dealing-with-aberrant-behaviors-in-patients (accessed April 1, 2019).
SOURCES: As presented by Jessica Merlin, November 29, 2018; Merlin et al., 2018.

term "abuse," providers should refer to a use disorder or addiction. In this alternative, less stigmatizing language, an "abuser," "addict," or "alcoholic" becomes a "person with a substance use disorder." Toxicology results are no longer either "clean" or "dirty," but "positive," "negative," or "unexpected." "Relapse" becomes a "return to use," and "bingeing" becomes "unhealthy," "excessive," or "heavy" use.

As to how to treat substance use disorder in patients with a serious illness, Merlin said the research is unclear on whether these patients should be treated in the same way that someone with a substance use disorder would be treated. "Should this be any different than how we treat addiction in anybody else?" asked Merlin. "The real answer is, we do not know." She added that what is known from the addiction literature is that treating substance use disorders saves lives, reduces high-risk behaviors, and improves quality of life, with the mainstream treatments being some combination of medications and psychosocial treatments.

Merlin emphasized that studies are needed that address whether buprenorphine or methadone works better in patients with pain and serious illness, whether methadone should be available in the provider's office and not just in methadone clinics, and what settings work best for delivering substance use disorder therapies, particularly given the shortage of substance use disorder specialists relative to the need. She would also like to see more research to identify how clinicians should balance compassion with managing a substance use disorder. Compassion, she reiterated, is not the same thing as prescribing opioids, and treating a substance use disorder is compassionate given that having a substance use disorder causes suffering.

Merlin explained that for people at the end of life, having a substance use disorder is a compulsion with negative consequences. She described these consequences as including increased patient suffering; increased stress and frustration for family members and caregivers, masking symptoms important for patient care; family concern over misuse of medication; reluctance by providers to offer adequate pain medications; poor patient compliance with treatment protocols; and decreased quality of life (Passik and Theobald, 2000).

In conclusion, Merlin emphasized that managing chronic pain and substance use disorder in individuals with serious illness is challenging, but it is also important and rewarding. "We are here today because we are thought leaders in these issues, so who better than us to find a way forward to improve care for these patients?" asked Merlin.

Discussion

Following the speakers' presentations, session moderator Judith Paice, director of the cancer pain program in the Division of Hematology-Oncology and research professor of medicine at the Northwestern University Feinberg School of Medicine, opened the discussion session. Paice noted that patients in methadone clinics in Chicago are being kicked out of the programs when they develop a serious illness because methadone clinic directors do not perceive they have the expertise to deal with these patients. This is causing a great deal of existential distress for the patients, and for the clinicians treating them for their serious illness.

Workshop participant Craig Blenderman commented that cancer pain and pain in patients with serious illness with a history of substance use disorder or high risk of opioid use disorder can be managed effectively with methadone or buprenorphine. He asked why the field does not advocate for this as a first-line strategy if there are no contraindications. Merlin replied that she agreed completely given that methadone and buprenorphine are evidence-based treatments. When she has a patient with chronic pain and an opioid use disorder, regardless of whether there is also a serious illness, she prescribes buprenorphine because she does not work in a licensed methadone clinic. Merlin pointed out that methadone for pain is dosed differently than methadone for opioid use disorder. However, if she sends a patient to a methadone clinic, someone has to have a conversation with the clinic staff member, who often does not feel comfortable prescribing methadone for pain. Merlin noted that research is needed that examines methadone use for pain in patients with serious illness as well as policy changes that bring methadone clinics into the health care system.

Daniel Alford of Boston University and Boston Medical Center reiterated that it is not permissible to prescribe methadone for treatment of an opioid use disorder outside of a federally licensed methadone clinic. Therefore, the prescribing physician has to be clear that a methadone prescription is for pain even though a person has a history of or is currently struggling with opioid use disorder. However, diagnosing an opioid use disorder in that patient and then continuing to prescribe methadone is illegal, even though it is appropriate clinically and pharmacologically.

Alford further noted that there is evidence showing that patients with a history of an opioid use disorder, whether active or in recovery, and whether on methadone, buprenorphine, or no medication, tend to have increased pain sensitivity compared with matched controls. Alford said,

There is anxiety associated with that, so there are things we do to reassure these patients that we understand that their sensitivity may be increased, but also that just because they have a history of a substance use disorder, we are not going to undertreat them, and we are actually going to be more aggressive. I think that goes a long way in helping some of these patients deal with their pain, realizing that we appreciate that they have a different experience.

Barbara Herbert from the Commonwealth Care Alliance asked Merlin to comment on how she deals with people who are in pain and may be in remission from an opioid use disorder, but who are self-medicating with alcohol or cannabis. Merlin replied that this is a common occurrence because substance use disorders are often polysubstance use disorders. When one of her patients with an opioid use disorder uses alcohol in a way that is risky or constitutes an alcohol use disorder, or uses cannabis, Merlin suggests a risk–benefit analysis and a direct conversation with the patient. Her main concern is that all of these substances are sedatives, so when she has someone on opioids who is also using alcohol, she tries hard to get them to be in recovery from alcohol. Regarding cannabis, her view is that the evidence base is still missing as far as its use in treating pain in conjunction with long-term opioid therapy. She stressed the importance of always weighing the risks and benefits of the substances the patient is taking.

Jeri Miller from the Office of End of Life Palliative Care Research at the National Institute of Nursing Research applauded Merlin for her candid remarks about the need for a contemporary knowledge base. Miller then pointed out that the National Institutes of Health (NIH) has had a funding announcement for several years called Mechanisms, Models, Measurement, and Management in Pain Research.[16] "We found over the years that we could not bring in individuals who are interested in pain and serious illness," she said. As a result, her institute launched two funding opportunity announcements that focus on symptom management, with one primary objective being to look at pain and how it interacts with behavioral and mental health issues, the family caregiver, and social determinants of health. She also mentioned that NIH, the U.S. Department of Defense, and the VA have an $81 million initiative looking at pain management and patient outcomes in real world, pragmatic settings using practical approaches. She then challenged the workshop participants to take advantage of those funding opportunities to produce the missing evidence.

---

[16] For more information, see https://grants.nih.gov/grants/guide/pa-files/PA-18-141.html (accessed January 23, 2019).

Heather Wargo, a patient advocate for patients such as those with chronic pancreatitis and interstitial cystitis, asked Merlin if any of her colleagues are studying whether long-term opioid use can help patients who do not have many treatment options. She also asked about research on patients being taken off opioids despite being in significant pain. Merlin remarked that Wargo's question raised the issue of a patient being taken off opioids due to opioid use disorder compared with being taken off due to insurance coverage or policy reasons. Merlin referred to Kertesz's earlier presentation in which he described the issue of engaging in shared decision making with a patient to develop a plan for tapering if that seems to be appropriate for a given patient. She noted there is little information on patient outcomes from patients who are "yanked off" opioids other than "disturbing anecdotes that are bubbling up to the surface." Kertesz commented that several abstracts have been presented at public meetings about people being discontinued from opioids and what the outcomes are, but those studies have not been peer reviewed yet. The literature "will be much more robust about a year from now," he said.

Kertesz then asked Merlin a question about another way of diagnosing opioid use disorder in which a provider will stop giving patients opioids by tapering slowly, and if the patient cannot cope, then the provider has "uncovered" opioid use disorder that warrants treatment. This method serves as a "stress test" of sorts, Kertesz explained. Merlin responded that she does not endorse the wholesale tapering of every patient off opioids and then watching to see if they have an opioid use disorder. She thinks tapering and diagnosing opioid use disorder are two different things. She stressed the importance of shared decision making. "Let's not give the whole population a stress test," she cautioned.

IMPACT OF POLICY AND REGULATORY RESPONSE TO THE OPIOID USE DISORDER EPIDEMIC ON THE CARE OF PEOPLE WITH SERIOUS ILLNESS

The fourth session of the workshop featured three presentations on how regulations and policies developed in response to the opioid use disorder epidemic are affecting the ways in which health care providers treat their patients with serious illness. Hemi Tewarson, director of the Health Division of the National Governors Association (NGA), reflected on her organization's work with states as they develop policies to address the opioid use disorder epidemic. Michael Botticelli, executive director of the Grayken

Center for Addiction at Boston Medical Center, discussed federal regulatory and policy responses based on his experience as director of the White House Office of National Drug Control Policy. He also described what is being done about these issues from the perspective of his current position in a large academic medical center. Trent Haywood, senior vice president and chief medical officer of the Blue Cross Blue Shield Association, provided a payer's perspective and discussed his organization's medical and pharmaceutical policy related to caring for people with serious illness.

State Policies Addressing the Opioid Use Disorder Epidemic

Tewarson noted that the opioid use disorder epidemic has been a top priority for the nation's governors since 2012, explaining that 22 new governors would be taking office in December 2018 and January 2019. While many of them will want to work on issues such as education and addressing the cost curve of health care, for example, the opioid use disorder epidemic is a challenge they will also need to address (see Figure 9). She pointed to the recent CDC data showing that life expectancy in the United States has declined because of opioid-related deaths. Tewarson stressed that more than 70,000 people died of a drug overdose in 2017, the highest number on record; the number of deaths due to drug overdose increased 9.6 percent from 2016 to 2017. Tewarson pointed out that overdose deaths from fentanyl and other synthetic opioids increased by 45 percent over that time period.

Governors, said Tewarson, are frustrated because they have what could be called "blunt" or non-personalized instruments to address this problem as the death rates continue to rise. As other speakers had noted, Tewarson said these blunt instruments, including prescription duration limits and dosage limits, are having unintended consequences for people with serious illness who need pain relief and palliative care.

Tewarson explained that in an effort to better address the opioid use disorder epidemic, NGA released a roadmap in 2016 with strategies for both opioids and heroin. This roadmap urged state leaders to assess their current capacity to deal with the epidemic and to identify evidence-based and promising practices they can deploy and evaluate not just in terms of reducing the number of prescriptions filled or overdose deaths, but also patient outcomes. She noted that in July 2016, the governors signed a compact stating that they would work to combat the opioid use disorder epidemic.

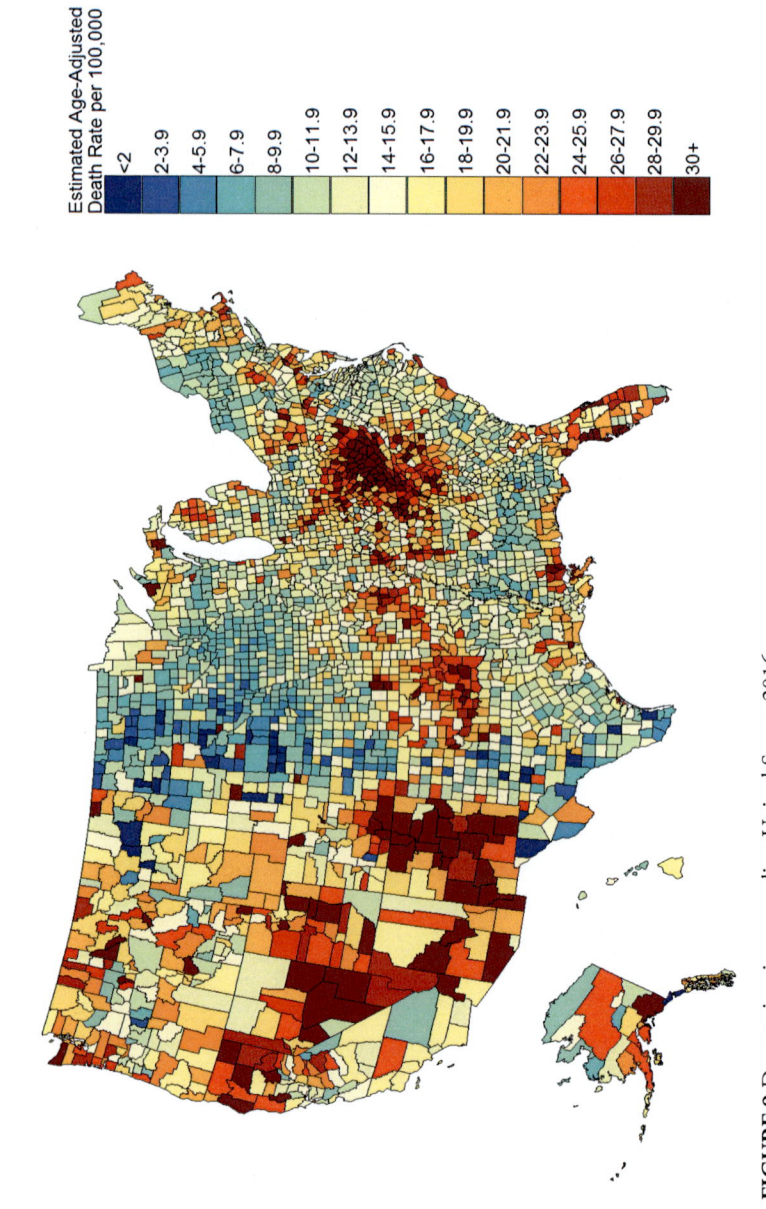

FIGURE 9 Drug poisoning mortality: United States, 2016.
SOURCES: As presented by Hemi Tewarson, November 29, 2018; Rossen et al., 2017.

In 2017, the governors reported on their progress. In Alaska, for example, then-Governor Bill Walker issued a public health disaster declaration, which authorized the state Department of Health and Social Services to issue a medical standing order that allows community groups, law enforcement, and members of the public to dispense and administer naloxone. In New Jersey, then-Governor Chris Christie called for and signed legislation requiring insurers to cover immediate access to treatment for substance use disorder, including inpatient, outpatient, and medication-assisted treatment (MAT) for up to 6 months, which made New Jersey the only state at the time to guarantee coverage.

Much of the activity at the state level, said Tewarson, has focused on reducing the flow of opioid prescriptions by limiting first-time prescriptions and promoting clinical guidelines for safe prescribing. States have also been working on transforming pain management by supporting and enhancing community-based collaboration and increasing non-opioid treatment benefits. They are also expanding access to MAT and Medicaid coverage of treatment services, including for those who are in prison, as well as building the workforce needed to provide treatment services.

Tewarson reiterated that state prescribing policies have been relatively blunt instruments. Fifteen states have set 7-day prescribing limits, for example, and four states have 3- to 4-day limits. Though all of these states have exceptions for people with chronic pain and cancer, as well as for those who are in palliative care, providers in these states are concerned about how to apply these exceptions. While her organization does not represent state legislatures, it conducted a scan of 45 states and identified 480 bills that aim to deal with the opioid use disorder epidemic.

NGA has developed a list of nine areas in which states should focus to find solutions to the opioid and substance use disorder crisis:

1. Sharing information.
2. Reducing heroin and illicit fentanyl availability and use.
3. Improving access to addiction treatment in rural areas.
4. Providing MAT for justice-involved populations.
5. Developing strategies to address infectious diseases related to substance use disorder.
6. Reducing the incidence of neonatal abstinence syndrome.
7. Leveraging state emergency powers to address the epidemic.
8. Using non-opioid pain management.
9. Coordinating state and local frameworks.

One example of how a state is improving access to addiction treatment in rural areas is New Mexico's Project Echo. This project is designed to increase workforce capacity exponentially, particularly among primary care physicians, and to provide best practice specialty care and reduce health disparities. The program's success at increasing access to addiction treatment in rural and underserved areas of the state has prompted other states to establish their own Project Echo initiatives.[17]

Massachusetts, said Tewarson, has been the model state for increasing MAT in prison populations and connecting those released from prison to services in their communities. Ohio, meanwhile, is leading efforts to reduce neonatal abstinence syndrome through its program that provides holistic care for pregnant women. She noted that the White House and HHS have taken an interest in this program. Tewarson's organization is now helping other states learn how to implement it. However, some states have laws that threaten to remove a child from a mother if she comes forward with a substance use disorder, so there is work that needs to be done to change those laws.

With regard to increasing access to non-opioid pain management therapies, NGA convened a roundtable to identify possible solutions, particularly regarding coverage policies, that will generate a white paper for state leaders. In the meantime, Ohio has already decided to have its Medicaid plan cover acupuncture and chiropractic services provided by licensed practitioners. South Dakota took the approach of increasing access to non-opioid therapies through Medicaid-eligible health homes. The goal was to provide centralized locations that could provide multiple services to individuals.

In closing, Tewarson reiterated comments made by others at the workshop that the policy exceptions states have carved out for patients with cancer and serious illness may not be working as intended. She noted, too, that states are working with a variety of partners to address all of the factors of pain using pharmacological and non-pharmacological treatment and to deliver ongoing provider education on appropriate prescribing of opioids and the potential for patient misuse.

---

[17] For more information, see https://echo.unm.edu (accessed March 6, 2019).

A Federal Perspective on Policies and Regulatory Approaches

Before launching into his presentation, Botticelli explained that not only was he the former director of National Drug Control Policy, but prior to that role he was Massachusetts's state director for Addiction Services, which he said gives him both federal and state perspectives. Moreover, he said that because patient experience is such a critical part of this conversation, he believed it was important to acknowledge that he is a person in long-term recovery from substance use disorder, so he also experiences this issue from that perspective. As someone who has straddled the world between science and politics for a very long time, he said that while some policies and programs are implemented based on rigorous scientific evidence, others are not, and in those instances the best to hope for is to mitigate the harm of bad policy. "The challenge as a policy maker and as a practitioner is that you cannot sit and do nothing while you wait for the accumulation of evidence," said Botticelli.

Botticelli explained that what he tried to do as a policy maker was to look at the causes of a problem, consider what the available evidence says is causing the problem, and then try to implement programs that address those causes. In his role with the federal government, one of the most frustrating aspects of his job was how often he was reacting to 2-year-old data that provide little real-time insights, both in terms of how well a policy is working as well as whether there are unintended consequences of that policy. In his opinion, accelerating the collection, analysis, and dissemination would help policy makers tremendously.

Turning to the federal response to the opioid use disorder epidemic, Botticelli highlighted the role that the Patient Protection and Affordable Care Act and Medicaid expansion have played in increasing access to treatment. "Having substance use disorder treatment as one of the 10 essential benefits was revolutionary in terms of people getting treatment," he said. In states hardest hit by the opioid use disorder epidemic, such as Kentucky and West Virginia, there were significant increases in treatment, and particularly MAT. In Dayton, Ohio, the mayor attributed Medicaid expansion in her state as one of the most significant reasons why her city has seen a 50 percent reduction in overdose deaths, noted Botticelli.

In 2011, prior to leaving his position in Massachusetts and joining the federal government, the administration released its prescription drug abuse prevention plan. This plan included four pillars:

1. The first pillar of the prescription drug abuse prevention plan focused on educating the public about prevention-related issues and physicians about safer opioid prescribing. The plan, said Botticelli, tried to promote a balanced view—one that did not just talk about reducing opioid prescribing, but also the individuals for whom it is appropriate to have access to opioid pain medications.
2. The second pillar of the plan was to create state-based PDMPs that would link data to electronic health records and share data among the states.
3. The third pillar focused on disposal as a means of curtailing diversion of legitimate prescriptions, one of the most significant sources of prescription drug misuse.
4. The fourth pillar concerned law enforcement, with efforts centered largely on shutting down the pill mills that Liebschutz had mentioned in her presentation. At one point, said Botticelli, Broward County, Florida, with its numerous pill mills, accounted for 50 percent of all U.S. opioid prescriptions.

Botticelli explained that when he became director of National Drug Control Policy, one of his interests was in expanding access to MAT, and the administration worked with Congress to take a number of significant actions in that regard. One act was to increase the allowable prescribing limit of buprenorphine pills. More significant was allowing nurse practitioners and physician assistants to prescribe buprenorphine.

Botticelli pointed out that he also worked with AMA to increase the number of physicians who apply for and get a waiver to prescribe buprenorphine. "Nearly 16 years after we had approved buprenorphine, we only have 4 percent of primary care providers in this country who have even gone through the waiver process, and probably only 50 percent of those actually treat people," said Botticelli. "We need to do a better job of promoting more widespread treatment for people with addiction. It has to be part of our strategy." Toward that end, Botticelli and his colleagues worked with the Substance Abuse and Mental Health Services Administration (SAMHSA) and CDC to expand MAT with a focus on providing resources to community health centers across the nation. The goal was to increase access in rural areas and to create better integration with primary care.

Another policy change that Botticelli considers important was mandating the creation of federal drug courts, as well as mandating that the courts and addiction treatment providers that receive federal dollars offer access to MAT. His office also promoted the expansion of naloxone distribution and Good Samaritan laws across the country.[18] This action was based on research showing that broader naloxone distribution in a community reduced overdose deaths (Kerensky and Walley, 2017).

One surprise accomplishment, said Botticelli, was convincing a conservative Congress to repeal the decades-old ban on using federal funding for sterile needle programs to combat the alarming rise of hepatitis C and HIV/AIDS in many communities affected by the opioid use disorder epidemic. The Office of National Drug Control Policy also worked to foster collaborative efforts between public health and public safety in high-intensity drug trafficking areas to increase information sharing.

Botticelli explained that some members of Congress believed that Medicaid expansion actually caused the opioid use disorder epidemic because it enabled more people to get more prescriptions for opioids. Several studies and articles, however, have proven this not to be true (Goodman-Bacon and Sandoe, 2017; Saloner et al., 2018; Venkataramani and Chatterjee, 2019), finding no difference in prescribing patterns before and after Medicaid expansion. What those studies did find were significant increases in prescriptions written for buprenorphine and naloxone. Another misconception, noted Botticelli, was that the focus on reducing opioid prescribing increased the use of heroin and fentanyl. Research has shown, however, that although that may be true for individual cases, it was not a population-level phenomenon, said Botticelli. He observed that the increase in heroin use and overdoses is likely a function of the progressive nature of substance use disorder and the fact that it is less expensive to buy heroin on the street than it is to buy prescription pain medication from a pharmacy.

Turning to the CDC guideline discussed by earlier speakers, Botticelli reiterated that the guideline has come with significant unintended consequences. In his view, the federal government needs to conduct an extensive evaluation of the guideline's impact, both positive and negative. Moreover, Botticelli and colleagues have called on Congress through a *New England Journal of Medicine* letter to revise the 50-year-old methadone regulations to allow for more integration into primary care (Samet et al., 2018). Botticelli noted that he received "pushback from the industry" and SAMHSA has indicated that it would not support the idea. Botticelli stressed that the nation urgently needs to consider regulatory reform for the

---

[18] For more information, see http://www.ncsl.org/research/civil-and-criminal-justice/drug-overdose-immunity-good-samaritan-laws.aspx (accessed March 6, 2019).

nation's methadone treatment programs. "We should not have to receive care in the worst part of town, and we should not have to go day after day after day for 6 months to be deemed compliant with treatment," he said. "We have seen with buprenorphine and now naltrexone, as well as from work in other countries, that we can do this in the context of primary care."

A Payer's Perspective on Policies to Address the Opioid Use Disorder Epidemic

In considering treatments for opioid use disorder, Trent Haywood pointed out that the key is having evidence to support payment decisions. "Where there is underlying evidence, there are opportunities to push solutions forward," said Haywood. "Where there is confusion as to what the underlying evidence is, you continue to have confusion about what the appropriate solution should be." He believes evidence is fundamentally critical to how his organization approaches solutions because this is not only a payment and policy issue, but a rudimentary learning system issue. He pointed to the importance and use of the "number needed to treat—number needed to harm" in determining if a treatment is covered.[19]

Haywood explained that he and his colleagues have access to rich patient data, and in combination with proprietary and public data, they can drill down beyond the county level to the block group level. Haywood shared that one thing he learned from this analysis was that the opioid use disorder epidemic in many areas resembles a communicable disease, which he called a shocking discovery until he considered it from a social practice standpoint. "That let us know that whatever solutions we bring to bear, it is not enough to look just inside the four walls of the hospital or clinic setting. Rather, you have to start to engage the community to understand what is occurring in those particular social practices," said Haywood.

Taking an evidence-based approach, Haywood and his colleagues found that with the exception of some serious illnesses, there was not much evidence supporting the use of opioids in the acute care setting. As a result, in May 2017, Blue Cross Blue Shield issued guidance that with the exception of certain serious illnesses, opioids should not be prescribed for first-line therapy. The challenge was to develop a learning system that allows for the exception for those with serious illness and provides this patient

---

[19] For more information, see https://www.cebm.net/2014/03/number-needed-to-treat-nnt (accessed March 6, 2019).

population with adequate support. The first step, noted Haywood, was to use medical claims and pharmacy information to develop an approach to identify patients with serious illness. Haywood explained that Blue Cross Blue Shield has also tried to exclude individuals with serious illness from prior authorization requirements and to automate the process as much as possible.

Noting the geographical variability surrounding coverage of non-traditional pain treatments such as acupuncture, Haywood stressed the need for evidence to support these non-opioid treatment alternatives as well as a mechanism for disseminating such evidence to all health care systems and payers.

In closing, Haywood stressed again the importance of creating a learning system to develop and disseminate the evidence to health care plans, patients, and society at large in an effort to address the opioid use disorder epidemic.

Discussion

Tulsky opened the discussion by asking the panelists to comment on what they think the greatest political pushbacks have been to enacting evidence-based policies in three areas of emphasis that Tewarson discussed: reducing prescriptions and access, increasing pain management, and expanding access for treatment for substance use disorder. Botticelli replied that regarding MAT, there is a great deal of pushback from treatment providers, state medical associations, and the recovery community, who support abstinence-based treatment. As a result, a significant number of people are reticent to go on medication. He noted that Narcotics Anonymous, which promotes a 12-step approach, does not support the use of medications. In his view, an unintended consequence of inaction around the opioid use disorder epidemic has led to some of the legislative mandates that have been put in place.

Haywood noted that some of the reluctance to turn to MAT can be traced to cultural differences. For example, in the U.S. South, where there are at-risk populations that would benefit from MAT, the social norms and practices of clinicians have led to a disconnect between need and the number of physicians willing to be certified as MAT providers.

Tewarson added that although there is evidence on the effectiveness of MAT for many of those with an opioid use disorder, there is no evidence on what works for people with serious illness or chronic pain and substance use disorder. In the meantime, until such data are available, she believes a more holistic approach of trying different things at the same time is one way to go.

Workshop participant Amy L. Small said speakers acknowledged that the CDC guideline has caused unintended consequences. She asked what each of the speakers would do to advocate for a massive revision or rescission of the CDC guideline. Haywood replied that he was not certain he agreed with the premise that the CDC guideline should be rescinded. Instead, he promoted the idea that evidence and data should be used to enhance or improve the guideline. Botticelli agreed with Haywood and added that the problem is not with the CDC guideline, but rather how it has been interpreted incorrectly. He then commented that it is likely there are other reasons that patients are having their access to opioids sharply curtailed and these need to be identified, too. "This is not just about the opioid [misuse] epidemic, and we have really got to get to root cause social issues," he said. There will be little progress, he added, if poverty, endemic racism, lack of educational and vocational opportunities, and social isolation are not part of the discussion.

Joanne Lynn of Altarum's Program to Improve Elder Care commented on Haywood's remark that the opioid use disorder epidemic resembles a communicable disease. Given that, she wondered if the conventional tools of public health, such as contact tracing and using public information, are being underused. To address the epidemic, Lynn said, there could be a focus on how substance use data are collected and used in public health systems. Haywood replied that he would be very supportive of trying to take CDC in that direction and that there are opportunities to do so. In fact, he said, if a public health model would be successful in helping to address the opioid use disorder epidemic, it could serve as a model for future public health epidemics. Botticelli said he has often wondered if recovery is contagious given the data from tobacco studies showing that if one person quits smoking, others in that proximity are more likely to quit smoking too. He also suggested that the same cascade of care model that has worked with HIV/AIDS, where progress was measured in terms of the percentage of people who get tested, the percentage who engage in care, the percentage who stay in care, and the percentage that reach zero viral load, might work with substance use disorder. In the case of substance use disorder, the corresponding metrics would be diagnosis rate, engagement rate, and some measure of recovery as the analogous marker to zero viral load.

Tewarson added that this epidemic is multifaceted. For example, there is a shortage of housing and community supportive services for those in recovery. States, she noted, have been experimenting with how to integrate the different services to best support those in recovery or who are trying to reach to that place. NGA has been pushing to have Congress address the barriers to sharing data included in the Confidentiality of Alcohol and Drug Abuse Patient Records, 42 CFR Part 2, which deals with the confidentiality of substance use disorder patient records.[20]

Workshop participant David Steinhorn from Children's National Medical Center wanted to reinforce Friedrichsdorf's message that one in five citizens is a pediatric patient. He worries about the trickle-down effect of adult policy influencing the pediatric community. "If these policies are too restricted for the benefit of adult patients, they are going to limit our ability to care for children," said Steinhorn. He said it is important that the pediatric agenda for prescribing opioids for children with advanced disease is separate from the adult agenda.

Alford asked the panelists to comment on why insurers stopped paying for multimodal comprehensive pain management programs, which had the effect of eliminating them, whereas interventions of specialty pain programs are paid for even though they are not evidence based. He also commented on the possibility of moving decision making on reimbursement away from needing robust evidence of efficacy, which will take time to generate, and instead looking at risk. Massage therapy, acupuncture, and cognitive behavioral therapies are not risky, for example. Haywood replied that reimbursement decisions are not traditionally based solely on the risk or lack thereof of a particular treatment. Insurers do not change the standard for evidence for each treatment. Only after the treatment has reached a certain level of evidence would payers look at comparative effectiveness and risk. From a state Medicaid perspective, said Tewarson, there is interest in determining how to cover these different types of treatments for different populations and under what circumstances.

Herbert commented that, even in cases where approaches such as physical therapy are effective, prior authorization requirements are onerous and complicate the lives of physicians tremendously. In her opinion, insurers have not stepped up to accept non-pharmacological interventions except by creating onerous prior authorizations. She then challenged Haywood, as he talks to other insurers, to figure out ways to incorporate

---

[20] This law generally requires a federally assisted substance use program to have a patient's consent before releasing information to others. It encourages people to seek treatment and reassures patient privacy (SAMHSA, 2018).

non-pharmacological approaches for treating pain. She noted that the providers of these approaches do not have the financial resources to conduct trials to generate evidence of effectiveness in a standard clinical trial setting. Haywood replied that the Patient-Centered Outcomes Research Institute is able to do that research without having to worry about the financial payback associated with a pharmacological therapy, and it should serve as the vehicle for doing such studies.

CARING FOR PEOPLE WITH SERIOUS ILLNESS IN THE CONTEXT OF THE OPIOID USE DISORDER EPIDEMIC: LESSONS TO INFORM POLICY AND PRACTICE

The workshop's final session offered the opportunity for five panelists, as well as the workshop attendees, to reflect on the lessons learned throughout the day and to chart a path forward. As an introduction to the final session, Dreyfus summarized the key themes he had heard throughout the day (see Box 2). Dreyfus noted that he did not hear any discussion about how changes to the reimbursement system, in terms of shifting from a fee-for-service approach to a value-based approach, can have a positive effect on the way in which substance use disorder treatments are delivered. He pointed out that a value-based approach relies on patient outcomes, regardless of what treatment modality the physician decides to use.

For the first panelist, Bob Twillman, executive director of the Academy of Integrative Pain Management and clinical associate professor at the University of Kansas School of Medicine, characterized that one of the most important things he heard was the need to address treatment of separate and co-occurring chronic pain and opioid use disorder. Another problem that he sees relates to mental health diagnoses. "How do we grapple with depression, anxiety, and posttraumatic stress," asked Twillman, and, "How do we grapple with adverse childhood experiences that contribute so much to these problems?" The difficulty, he said, is dealing with all three of these problems at the same time, and the answer to him is to pay attention to the whole patient, something that those who work in palliative care know better than anyone. "You have to pay attention to what is going on with the patient biologically, psychologically, socially, and spiritually to understand what is happening, and to find the right solutions," he said.

Jessica Nickel, founder, president, and chief executive officer of the Addiction Policy Forum, began her comments by noting that the Addiction Policy Forum is building a patient advocacy organization for the

> **BOX 2**
> **Summary of Key Themes Raised at the Workshop**
>
> - The opioid use disorder epidemic continues to claim a large number of lives—70,000 drug overdose deaths in 2017 alone—largely as a result of the increasing availability of powerful synthetic opioids such as fentanyl (NIDA, 2019).
> - Clinicians, patients, and families, especially families of color, struggle with accessing appropriate prescriptions for opioids for a number of reasons.
> - Clinicians face frustrations and moral distress when prescribing opioids due to hospital and pharmacy supply issues, burdensome policy requirements, and misinterpreted guidelines.
> - There is a huge knowledge gap regarding treating patients with co-occurring substance use disorder and pain.
> - There are deep systemic issues at the root of the tension between addressing the opioid use disorder epidemic and ensuring access to opioids for people who rely on them to manage their pain.
> - Stigma around addiction and behavioral health issues and limited availability of treatment programs have the effect of reducing access to effective treatment.
> - The fragmentation between the traditional medical care delivery system and the system for delivering substance use and mental health care services limits access to effective treatment.
> - There are social determinants of health contributing to the opioid use disorder epidemic.
> - Among the challenges to making greater use of alternatives to opioids is the lack of insurance coverage for these alternatives and a lack of non-opioid pain medications.
> - Research is needed to address gaps in evidence to support various pharmacologic and non-pharmacologic approaches to treating substance use disorder.
> - More health care providers need additional training on these topics.
> - Steps are being taken to expand access to substance use disorder treatment.
>
> SOURCE: As presented by Andrew Dreyfus, November 29, 2018.

patients and families struggling with substance use disorder. "This is a family disease—it feels like it hits your whole family—so bringing [patients and families] together and helping to navigate a new path is our mission," she explained. She pointed out that one concern she has after listening to the day's presentations and discussions is that one patient group is going to be pitted against another, and she called for looking at these issues from a broader perspective to avoid unintended consequences and oversimplification of complex problems.

Addiction is complicated, she said, and oversimplifying the problem leads to trouble. "We tend to play whack-a-mole with the drug du jour," said Nickel, noting that first the drug of concern was heroin, then it became cocaine, then crack cocaine, methamphetamine, prescription painkillers, and now synthetic opioids. The reality is the nation has a problem with substance use disorders in general and that most people with a substance use disorder have a problem with polydrug use. Although this problem starts in the doctor's exam room, she said, that is not where addiction truly begins. "The root causes are more complicated than that and takes more people at the table to fix it," said Nickel.

Nickel believes the root cause has two components. The first is that social norms are changing in the wrong direction. Some 15 million of the 20 million people struggling with a substance use disorder are dealing with an alcohol use disorder, and cultural norms around alcohol use do not address the situation (HHS, 2016). She reminded the workshop audience that substance use disorders typically begin in adolescence, and should be considered an adolescent brain disorder. Unfortunately, substance use disorders, for the most part, are treated in adulthood. "This is one of the only diseases that we wait for it to get worse before we intervene," said Nickel. She pointed out "what needs to happen is for there to be widespread acceptance among the public that substance use disorder is a health condition and it deserves a health care response."

She further noted the need for a better understanding of the role that trauma, particularly adverse childhood events and exposure to intergenerational substance use disorder, play in determining the risk of developing a substance use disorder. Moreover, greater understanding of the role of genetic predisposition is needed. In her experience, when people tell her they are reluctant to use an opioid because they might develop a substance use disorder, she asks them if substance use disorders run in the family and, if so, when they first started using alcohol, cannabis, or tobacco. The age of initiation is important, Nickel explained, due to brain development, which plays a role in the likelihood of the development of substance use disorder regardless of whether the brain is exposed to alcohol, cannabis, or another drug.

Another item on her organization's "wish list" is to integrate substance use disorder treatment into mainstream health care so that people do not have to uproot their lives and spend 28 days and thousands of dollars at a far-away treatment facility. "We need to find physicians who are going to help us manage a chronic condition that requires help for years, not 28 days, to manage," said Nickel.

Nickel also emphasized the importance of increasing prevention efforts, given that substance use disorder is a preventable illness. She explained that prevention is about delaying the age of onset, which means providing pediatricians and primary care physicians with the knowledge to teach parents and their adolescent patients how to protect themselves from this illness. Early detection and intervention must become part of the effort to solve the problem of substance use disorder, she said. "We do not wait for Stage IV before we treat cancer and we do not wait post-amputation before we initiate treatment for diabetes, so why is it that our culture distances itself or waits for the worst possible thing to happen when our patients are struggling with a substance use disorder?" she asked.

Alford stressed the need to better educate physicians about how to manage pain with modalities other than opioids, as well as to increase reimbursement for those modalities. The problem is that education is a slow process in health care. He noted that FDA's Risk Evaluation and Mitigation Strategy for opioids, which started in 2013, has completed more than 1,000 training programs and trained nearly 400,000 health care professionals nationwide. Education, he said, can be a finely tuned approach to individualizing care, as opposed to some of the blunt policy and regulatory instruments. "I believe that education has the potential benefit of reducing overprescribing while maintaining access to care for our patients," said Alford.

Alford explained that he has given a great deal of thought to why health care professionals have not been educated about chronic pain and substance use disorders, both of which are common, and opioids, which have been around for years. He believes the problem is that most academic medical centers do not have a department or center for substance use disorders or pain that can advocate for including those subjects in the curriculum. A key challenge is finding a way to train everyone at the same time. Alford explained that if training is provided only to medical students, it is not likely to be effective because once those students begin their rotations, they will see that experienced practitioners deal with pain and substance use disorder in different ways due to the lack of education and evidence to support one approach over another.

Alford pointed out that another challenge has to do with the subjective nature of pain, quality of life, and function and the difficulty measuring them in a meaningful way. This underscores the need to individualize care, which makes training that much more difficult because there is not some well-developed algorithm that will apply to all patients with pain. In Alford's view, the field needs to push the risk–benefit framework to the best of its ability while knowing that both the benefits and risks are subjective. Training needs to focus on identifying the nuances of deciding how much out-of-control behavior is enough to say a person has run into trouble and may have a substance use disorder, for example. The only way those undergoing training will learn that is to work with patients and actually have the difficult conversations with them about these complicated issues.

One controversy regarding such training is whether it should be mandatory. Alford said he would argue that everyone who is treating patients should be competent in how to assess and manage pain, prescribe opioids safely, and assess and manage opioid use disorders. He admitted that measuring competency at a national level will be challenging, but not beyond solving. He also noted that training cannot just be about prescriber education, but must include the entire health care team.

Reacting to Alford's remarks, Dreyfus pointed out that everything Alford said about the need for training and education around substance use disorder and pain management also applies to the care of people with serious illness.

Patrice Harris, president-elect of AMA and adjunct professor of psychology and behavioral sciences at Emory University, has chaired AMA's Opioid Task Force since 2014, and noted that the task force was convened to amplify what physicians were already doing in this area and to look at ways AMA could coordinate its efforts both within the profession and in partnership with other organizations. She then explained that the issues she hears from the public have to do with the lack of access to appropriate pain care, and the ways in which people in pain are stigmatized. One lesson she learned from the workshop is the need to be curious about a proposed intervention and to think about what the unintended consequences might be before acting. While acknowledging that there is a great deal of research needed, she said that where there is evidence, an intervention should be used, and where the evidence does not yet exist, admit it and then commit to evaluating an intervention. "I think we have the unintended consequences that we have because of a lack of commitment to evaluate some of the interventions that have been proposed and actually mandated," said Harris.

Harris then commented on the importance of challenging assumptions about individuals who have a substance use disorder, for example, and to recognize the implicit biases that come into play when treating someone with a substance use disorder. "That gets back to the science and the evidence and making sure we have the intellectual curiosity, but also the intellectual honesty, as we address these issues," said Harris.

To conclude her remarks, Harris briefly described the six recommendations that the Opioid Task Force developed for physicians:

1. Physicians should use their state's PDMP as a data tool.
2. Everyone should consider proposed therapies in a broader context. For example, it is easy to tell a patient to try physical therapy instead of opioids, but going to physical therapy requires transportation, time off work, arranging child care, and copays.
3. Physicians should enhance their education and training specific to their specialty or role in the health care system.
4. The issue of stigma should be elevated as well as the ways in which it affects those who have chronic pain or a substance use disorder.
5. Comprehensive treatments should be available for patients with pain and a substance use disorder.
6. The public should be able to access safe storage and disposal of opioids, as well as naltrexone.

Keith Humphreys, the Esther Ting Memorial Professor at Stanford University and senior research career scientist at the VA, said he hears people grappling with the fact that this is a dilemma, not a problem. Problems have clear solutions, he said, using cholera as an example. Cleaning the local water supply eliminates cholera and the issue is addressed, he said, but opioids are different. Noting that he worked in hospice care for 9 years, he pointed out that hospice care without opioids would be a horror. "No one has to convince me how incredible these medications are and how lucky we are to have them," said Humphreys. At the same time, he is a native of West Virginia and his state is being destroyed by opioid misuse, and that makes this a dilemma. What is important, he said, is not to be pro-opioid or anti-opioid, but pro-patient and to consider that there will be different solutions for each patient.

Humphreys emphasized that Americans need to have some respect and compassion for those who become addicted to their pain medication.

"These are our neighbors, our friends, our family, and they are human beings worthy of respect," said Humphreys. Too often, he said, "people call pain patients whiny, complaining [that] 'they need to buck up.'" He views that attitude as degrading and creates an environment where it is impossible to think clearly because everyone is understandably hurt and angry. He noted that experimental social psychologists have demonstrated that hurt and anger cause people to think in black and white and to come up with extreme solutions. "We need to grasp this dilemma and have respect and compassion for one another," said Humphreys.

Nuance, which is often in short supply in the policy world, is also needed, said Humphreys. While people argue about whether there are too many or too few opioids prescribed for people in pain, getting down to specifics can lead to places where agreement can be reached. As an example, Humphreys predicted that everyone would agree that 40 percent of people who go to the emergency department in Arkansas with a sprained ankle do not need to leave with a prescription for 30 Vicodin pills. "That is a place where we can cut back without hurting any chronic pain patient," said Humphreys, "and if that is your child getting that Vicodin, as a parent you are absolutely delighted at that reduction."

Humphreys referred to work by one of his graduate students modeling the health benefits and harms of public policy responses to the opioid use disorder epidemic (Pitt et al., 2018). This modeling work showed that "giving access to naloxone hurts nobody, helps everybody." Similarly, "expanding quality treatments for addition hurts nobody and helps everybody." Those are things, he said, that the field can rally around.

Discussion

To start the discussion, Dreyfus asked the panel for other ideas that the field could rally around to solve the dilemma Humphreys described. Twillman replied that he is always intrigued when he hears a payer say there is not enough evidence to cover non-pharmacological therapies for substance use disorder, when from his perspective, there is only low to moderate quality evidence that any therapy for pain—including opioid therapy—makes a moderate degree of difference over the short term. In fact, he noted, the Agency for Healthcare Research and Quality released a systematic review of non-pharmacological treatments for chronic pain and concluded that certain non-pharmacological therapies do show evidence of being effective for certain types of chronic pain (Skelly et al., 2018). "We have to get past the point of saying we have to have perfect evidence for everything before we decide to cover it, because if we wait for the evidence, we are never going to cover anything," said Twillman. His request, then, is for the field to push payers to be more specific about what they require and how they expect the field to get the type of evidence they want. He also proposed that payers might want to help the field establish demonstration projects to get the evidence they want. In his opinion, the field needs to "ramp up the volume" to payers to convince them that these other treatments are needed; if not, opioids will continue to be the only option.

Nickel's suggestion was for the field to help educate providers and patients on what risks looks like and what the risk factors truly are. She noted that better history taking, particularly regarding family history of substance or alcohol use disorder, could help identify potential risks and prevent substance use disorder from developing in the first place, though she acknowledged that more research is needed.

Alford, returning to his earlier comments, called for an investment in multidisciplinary faculty development across specialties given there is a limited number of board-certified pain specialists and substance use disorder specialists. He also proposed creating a clearinghouse for all of the educational materials that organizations such as CDC, FDA, AMA, the American College of Physicians, and many specialty societies have produced. Harris noted that AMA has a clearinghouse of all the information states and specialists have submitted on its Opioid Task Force microsite,[21] and that SAMHSA also has compiled resources.[22]

Harris then said she would like to add eliminating barriers to MAT to the list that Humphreys started. This would include eliminating the need for prior approvals for those who have insurance, providing appropriate reimbursement for individuals covered by Medicaid or Medicare, and eliminating copays for MATs, as has been done for methadone.

Humphreys added one more item to the list, which is to stop thinking of the current state as a crisis, because a crisis implies paying attention for a few years and then moving on to something else. "There has never been a time in the United States when addiction did not kill many people and disable many people, so it's not going to be solved by a 2-year grant to the

---

[21] For more information, see https://www.ama-assn.org/delivering-care/opioids/reversing-opioid-epidemic (accessed January 25, 2019).

[22] For more information, see https://www.samhsa.gov/homelessness-programs-resources/hpr-resources/useful-resources-opioid-overdose-prevention (accessed January 25, 2019).

states," said Humphreys. What needs to happen, he said, is for substance use disorder and its treatments to be incorporated into the structure of medicine. In the United States, that means building it into the financing of medicine by getting CMS to change reimbursements under Medicaid and Medicare so that substance use disorder treatments are reimbursed at the same level as cancer and heart disease, Humphreys explained.

Amy Melnick of the National Coalition for Hospice and Palliative Care informed the panelists that there were many pain patients viewing the workshop webcast online, and one posed a question on behalf of a patient with ankylosing spondylitis—arthritis that can affect the spine. The patient asked if the panelists were aware that pain management clinics will kick people out of their programs if CBD or another cannabis-related substance is found in routine urinalysis, even in states where medical or recreational cannabis is legal. The patient also asked if the workshop's discussions could lead to advocacy for change regarding cannabis use for pain. Twillman replied that the issue of medical marijuana, and CBD in particular, is challenging. He explained that his organization has asked him to develop a position statement, but because of the state of the science, he is not in a position to do so. His concern is that stating today that medical marijuana is useful for pain treatment without sufficient evidence might be premature if, 10 years from now, it turns out there is a huge problem with cannabis addiction. "We need to continue to figure out how this works for people, for whom it works, why it works, and how best to deliver care," said Twillman.

Anne Fuqua from the Alliance for the Treatment of Intractable Pain commented that she has been on 1,000 morphine milligram equivalents for more than a decade, fortunately without side effects, and her quality of life has benefitted as a result. She acknowledged that doses that high are not appropriate for most people, and that such doses often do cause significant side effects, but that tapering patients who truly benefit from higher doses can degrade their quality of life. She then recounted that when her physician of 9 years closed his pain management clinic, what followed was the worst experience of her life. While she has been able to find a physician who would prescribe high-dose opioid therapy, it requires her to travel from Alabama, where she lives, to California every 3 months, at great cost. She asked the panelists how health care providers can be enabled to be pro-patient and ensure that long-term patients who are stable on high doses continue to have access to those medications.

Harris responded that Fuqua's experience illustrates the importance of individualized care and looking at patients, not doses. She noted that AMA has been steadfast in its commitment that decisions regarding treatment should be between the patient and their physician despite all the external disincentives to do so. She acknowledged that the threat of a DEA action and loss of license to practice will certainly lead a physician to change prescribing habits. "Doctors should not have to be afraid," said Harris. Dreyfus added that there needs to be more team-based care in a team that includes the patient and the family.

Friedrichsdorf asked the panelists for their ideas on how to better advocate for children who have serious illness and pain. Nickel said one key to doing better for children is follow Humphreys's proposal to bring substance use disorders into the mainstream of medical practice and embed treatment of these disorders within the nation's health care system. Pediatricians, she added, need to be at the table when developing solutions. Harris noted that AMA's new pain task force will address the pediatric population and that the American Academy of Pediatrics is represented on the Opioid Task Force (AMA, n.d.). Dreyfus pointed out that Massachusetts's efforts include working on prevention in the state's middle schools.

Benita Talati, a patient with Ehlers-Danlos Syndrome, asked how serious illness is defined beyond palliative care and cancer pain. She noted that there are people who live with chronic pain, but are not cancer patients or on palliative care, who have lost access to opioid medications or who have never been prescribed them. Twillman replied that the core issue is suffering, and from his perspective, anyone suffering with pain has a serious illness. Talati replied that the problem is that insurance will often not cover certain pain management approaches. Dreyfus commented that the Roundtable on Quality Care for People with Serious Illness is trying to address these issues through activities such as this public workshop. The idea for the workshop, he explained, grew out of the broad recognition that there are millions of patients struggling with chronic illness and chronic pain who are caught between the blunt responses to the opioid use disorder epidemic and the need to manage pain.

Wargo, who suffers from incurable pancreatic and biliary disease and could not function without her high-dose opioid therapy, noted that while there were more than 70,000 opioid-related deaths, largely from fentanyl, the number of deaths from prescribed opioids fell by 16 percent in 2017 from 2016. Her suggestion was to educate providers to do a better job of securing their opioid medications and limit the number of short-term prescriptions they are writing.

Liebschutz observed that people who have chronic pain or a substance use disorder live with it all day, every day, but they are only within the four walls of the health care system for 20 minutes every once in a while. Therefore, she said, when thinking about solutions, those solutions should be integrated into a patient's life and the patient's community needs to be brought into the solution. She then posed the question of how technology and the ubiquity of smartphones might factor into solutions to help people with chronic pain. Humphreys called that a great idea and noted that when one hospital tried to link patients to groups such as Alcoholics Anonymous and Narcotics Anonymous, it found that in the year after treatment those patients made far less use of mental health services and were in better health overall. To him, this shows the power of connectedness, which is something that online networks can promote. Dreyfus added that there had not been any discussion so far about the role of recovery coaches, but they will be an important piece of future treatment systems that health plans should cover.

Amy Berman of The John A. Hartford Foundation recounted a conversation she had with someone who pointed out that when patients first start on opioid therapy, they may need to go back repeatedly in the first month or so to have the dose adjusted. The multiple prescriptions they receive as a result of these adjustments can cause them to be dropped by their pharmacies because of the blunt tools that health plans use in response to the opioid use disorder epidemic. She asked the panelists for their ideas on how to ameliorate the effects of those blunt tools. Harris said sharing those stories is important, and AMA has asked physicians and patients to send in these stories where patients have been "unceremoniously dumped at pharmacies." She also recommended sharing these stories with state insurance authorities. Harris said that AMA will use these stories to advocate for change at the state and federal levels and with payers and pharmacies engaging in this behavior.

Twillman said it would help if partial fills of prescriptions were allowed, which was included in legislation passed several years ago. The DEA, however, has not yet written the regulations to allow that to happen despite pressure from Congress to do so. Alford agreed that allowing for partial fills would help and added that preauthorization requirements can make it difficult to try different medications or to rotate medications to avoid escalating doses. Nickel then commented on the importance of addressing the societal stigma that patients with chronic pain are now sharing with those who have substance use disorders. The way to do this, she said, is to educate the nation that chronic pain, as well as substance use disorder, is a health condition. Nickel noted that 49 percent of Americans believe chronic pain and substance use disorder are moral failings.

Humphreys commented that scientific studies are about finding the average effect of an intervention, but people are individuals, not averages. The hard part of a physician's job, then, is to say that the average does not apply to a particular patient and not surrender autonomy to a guideline, which he said is not the same as a mandate.

Kertesz raised the issue of how the health care community at large defines serious illness. He questioned what can and should be considered "serious" and therefore receive insurance coverage, as well as opioid therapy. In his view, payers and health care providers are "not great" at describing multidimensional illnesses. He recommended including nurses, rehabilitation specialists, "and maybe anthropologists" in the conversation on how to describe this type of suffering.

Zachary Sager, a psychiatrist and palliative care physician in Boston, asked the panelists to comment on the need to teach providers about trauma-informed care given that he has never seen anyone with either a serious illness or a substance use disorder who has not been traumatized. He asked what is being done in education and training to teach about trauma-informed care. Harris replied that this is an issue that needs to be elevated. Trauma, she pointed out, is also involved in heart disease, diabetes, and other chronic illnesses. At the same time, it is important to consider what this would mean for policy, particularly concerning how to address trauma in early childhood education.

Alford pointed that part of the problem with pain is that physicians are worried about treating acute pain as if it is chronic pain, and that writing one prescription for an opioid is going to result in addiction or overdose. "We need to be smart about this," said Alford. "If a person has terrible acute pain, providing a day or two of an opioid is not going to result in addiction, and it might allow that person to go to physical therapy or return to work." What should not happen, he said, is writing a prescription for a 30-day supply for someone who has acute pain. The situation for a person with chronic pain is different and needs to be managed as a chronic, multidimensional problem.

Shari Ling of CMS remarked that the day's presentations and discussions served as a poignant reminder of how the nation's health care system has been challenging for the very people it is intended to serve. In thinking about opportunities that everyone can act on, she said the transition to a value-focused system affords the opportunity to deliver person-centered care, which would include when a person is not a patient. To her, that means having clinicians and patients co-designing high-quality care plans.

Smith added that there needs to be a way of ensuring that a care plan is in fact a good one and not just a means of checking a box related to providing value-based care. Dreyfus said the key there is to focus on outcomes, not processes; just as it is important to stop counting pills and look at patient outcomes. Twillman agreed, stating that often stakeholders "confuse quality with fewer opioid pills being prescribed." Nickel also noted that what struck her among the suggestions and priorities she heard is the need to collaborate for better patient outcomes for those individuals with chronic pain and those with substance use disorders.

Alford commented on the experience of an English professor who is in chronic pain and is on long-term opioid therapy who wrote about his rather humiliating experiences every time he refills his prescription (Unger, 2017). "We can try to estimate what the patient experience is around opioids and pain and addiction, but actually to hear from the patient's experience from the minute they walk in the door to the minute they leave I think addresses the whole issue around stigma and is a perspective that we cannot understand until we talk to them," he said.

Harris reminded the workshop participants that there is hope for all patients who have substance use disorders and those who suffer with chronic pain, if patients are put at the center of care, if care plans are crafted for the individual, and if every care plan considers potential unintended consequences. She noted that there are treatment paradigms for both substance use disorder and chronic pain that are working well, so the challenge is to disseminate information about those programs. Humphreys agreed there is reason to hope that these issues can be addressed, using the progress made with HIV/AIDS as an example of how a problem thought to be intractable can be solved. "If we are willing to work together and willing to invest the resources, we can save many, many lives, we can improve public health, we can improve pain management, and we can reduce addiction at the same time," said Humphreys.

In closing the final discussion, Tulsky offered three observations. First, many of the issues that were discussed during the workshop have been addressed in reports from the National Academies, including the IOM report *Relieving Pain in America* (IOM, 2011). In his view, the field has actually generated a great deal of knowledge and the issue now lies more in dissemination and implementation. Second, he emphasized the need for more communication between those in the chronic pain and serious illness world, and those in the substance use disorders field. From his perspective as a clinician, it appears that many of the competencies required of these two fields are analogous and that they both need to be patient centered.

Tulsky's final point focused on the need to change the public narrative and language used to talk about serious illness, chronic pain, and substance use disorders that undercut the ability for good outcomes. In his opinion, there is far more agreement than disagreement in these fields and the ways in which these issues are framed might be getting in the way of more constructive efforts to address this dilemma.

As a closing comment, Dreyfus said that he believes some of the conflicts discussed during the day represent conflicts between population health interventions and the individual needs of patients. "We have to try our best to resolve those conflicts," said Dreyfus.

REFERENCES

Alió, J. L., and J. Pikkel. 2014. Multifocal intraocular lenses: Neuroadaptation. *Multifocal Intraocular Lenses* 47–52.

AMA (American Medical Association). *Reversing the opioid epidemic.* https://www.ama-assn.org/delivering-care/opioids/reversing-opioid-epidemic (accessed February 1, 2019).

Anand, K. J., B. A. Barton, N. McIntosh, H. Lagercrantz, E. Pelausa, T. E. Young, and R. Vasa. 1999. Analgesia and sedation in preterm neonates who require ventilatory support: Results from the NOPAIN trial. Neonatal outcome and prolonged analgesia in neonates. *Archives of Pediatrics & Adolescent Medicine* 153(4):331–338.

APA (American Psychiatric Association). 2013. *Diagnostic and statistical manual of mental disorders.* Washington, DC: American Psychiatric Association.

Arthur, J. A., T. Edwards, Z. Lu, S. Reddy, D. Hui, J. Wu, D. Liu, J. L. Williams, and E. Bruera. 2016. Frequency, predictors, and outcomes of urine drug testing among patients with advanced cancer on chronic opioid therapy at an outpatient supportive care clinic. *Cancer* 122(23):3732–3739.

ASHP (American Society of Health–System Pharmacists). 2018. *Injectable opioid survey report: Impact of injectable opioid shortage and update on small-volume parenteral solution supplies.* https://www.ashp.org/Drug-Shortages/Shortage-Resources/Injectable-Opioid-Survey-Report (accessed March 19, 2019).

Beyer, J. E., D. E. DeGood, L. C. Ashley, and G. A. Russell. 1983. Patterns of postoperative analgesic use with adults and children following cardiac surgery. *Pain* 17(1):71–81.

Broome, M. E., A. Richtsmeier, V. Maikler, and M. Alexander. 1996. Pediatric pain practices: A national survey of health professionals. *Journal of Pain Symptom Management* 11(5):312–320.

Bruera, E. 2018. Parenteral opioid shortage—treating pain during the opioid-overdose epidemic. *New England Journal of Medicine* 379(7):601–603.

Cancino, A. 2016. *More grandparents raising their grandchildren.* https://www.pbs.org/newshour/nation/more-grandparents-raising-their-grandchildren (accessed February 15, 2019).

Case, A., and A. Deaton. 2015. Rising morbidity and mortality in midlife among white non-Hispanic Americans in the 21st century. *Proceedings of the National Academy of Sciences of the United States of America* 112(49):15078–15083.

CDC (Centers for Disease Control and Prevention). 2018. Understanding the epidemic. https://www.cdc.gov/drugoverdose/epidemic/index.html (accessed February 22, 2019).

Compton, W. M., and N. D. Volkow. 2006. Major increases in opioid analgesic abuse in the United States: Concerns and strategies. *Drug Alcohol Dependence* 81(2):103–107.

Compton, W. M., C. M. Jones, and G. T. Baldwin. 2016. Relationship between nonmedical prescription-opioid use and heroin use. *New England Journal of Medicine* 374(2):154–163.

Dabbs, J. 2019. Prescription Drug Monitoring Passes Missouri House, Here's How Lake-Area Reps Voted. *Lake Expo*. https://www.lakeexpo.com/news/politics/prescription-drug-monitoring-passes-missouri-house-here-s-how-lake/article_01c6f70e-2f13-11e9-a4ef-e32b161e6f9c.html (accessed March 26, 2019).

Demidenko, M. I., S. K. Dobscha, B. J. Morasco, T. H. A. Meath, M. A. Ilgen, and T. I. Lovejoy. 2017. Suicidal ideation and suicidal self-directed violence following clinician-initiated prescription opioid discontinuation among long-term opioid users. *General Hospital Psychiatry* 47:29–35.

Dowell, D., T. M. Haegerich, and R. Chou. 2016. CDC guideline for prescribing opioids for chronic pain—United States, 2016. *Morbidity and Mortality Weekly Report: Recommendations and Reports* 65(1):1–49.

Eland, J. M., and J. E. Anderson. 1977. The experience of pain in children. In *Pain: A source book for nurses and other health care professionals*, edited by A. Jacox. Boston, MA: Little Brown & Co. Pp. 453–478.

Ellis, J. A., B. V. O'Connor, M. Cappelli, J. T. Goodman, R. Blouin, and C. W. Reid. 2002. Pain in hospitalized pediatric patients: How are we doing? *The Clinical Journal of Pain* 18(4):262–269.

Feudtner, C., R. M. Hays, G. Haynes, J. R. Geyer, J. M. Neff, and T. D. Koepsell. 2001. Deaths attributed to pediatric complex chronic conditions: National trends and implications for supportive care services. *Pediatrics* 107(6):e99.

Frank, J. W., T. I. Lovejoy, W. C. Becker, B. J. Morasco, C. J. Koenig, L. Hoffecker, H. R. Dischinger, S. K. Dobscha, and E. E. Krebs. 2017. Patient outcomes in dose reduction or discontinuation of long-term opioid therapy: A systematic review. *Annals of Internal Medicine* 167(3):181–191.

Friedrichsdorf, S. J. 2017. Contemporary pediatric palliative care: Myths and barriers to integration into clinical care. *Current Pediatric Reviews* 13(1):8–12.

Friedrichsdorf, S. J., A. Postier, D. Eull, C. Weidner, L. Foster, M. Gilbert, and F. Campbell. 2015. Pain outcomes in a US children's hospital: A prospective cross-sectional survey. *Hospital Pediatrics* 5(1):18–26.

Friedrichsdorf, S. J, J. Giordano, K. D. Dakojo, A. Warmuth, C. Daughtry, and C. A. Schulz. 2016. Chronic pain in children and adolescents: Diagnosis and treatment of primary pain disorders in head, abdomen, muscles and joints. *Children (Basel)* 3(4):42.

Giusti, R., M. Mazzotta, L. Verna, I. Sperduti, F. R. Di Pietro, P. Marchetti, and G. Porzio. 2019. The incidence of alcoholism in patients with advanced cancer receiving active treatment in two tertiary care centers in Italy. *Alcohol and Alcoholism* 54(1):47–50.

Goodman-Bacon, A., and E. Sandoe. 2017. Did Medicaid expansion cause the opioid epidemic? There's little evidence that it did. In *Health Affairs blog: Following the ACA*. Bethesda, MD: Health Affairs.

Goyal, M. K., N. Kuppermann, S. D. Cleary, S. J. Teach, and J. M. Chamberlain. 2015. Racial disparities in pain management of children with appendicitis in emergency departments. *JAMA Pediatrics* 169(11):996–1002.

Green, C. R., S. K. Ndao-Brumblay, B. West, and T. Washington. 2005. Differences in prescription opioid analgesic availability: Comparing minority and white pharmacies across Michigan. *The Journal of Pain* 6(10):689–699.

HHS (U.S. Department of Health and Human Services). 2016. *Facing addiction in America: The Surgeon General's report on alcohol, drugs and health*. https://addiction.surgeongeneral.gov/sites/default/files/executive-summary.pdf (accessed April 1, 2019).

Ho, P., and R. Rosenheck. 2018. Substance use disorder among current cancer patients: Rates and correlates nationally in the Department of Veterans Affairs. *Psychosomatics* 59(3):267–276.

Interagency Pain Research Coordinating Committee. 2016. *National pain strategy*. Bethesda, MD: National Institutes of Health.

IOM (Institute of Medicine). 2011. *Relieving pain in America: A blueprint for transforming prevention, care, education, and research*. Washington, DC: The National Academies Press.

IOM. 2015. *Dying in America: Improving quality and honoring individual preferences near the end of life*. Washington, DC: The National Academies Press.

Jick, H., O. S. Miettinen, S. Shapiro, G. P. Lewis, V. Siskind, and D. Slone. 1970. Comprehensive drug surveillance. *JAMA* 213(9):1455–1460.

Kaiser Family Foundation. 1999. *Race, ethnicity & medical care: A survey of public perceptions and experiences*. San Francisco, CA: Kaiser Family Foundation.

Kaiser Family Foundation. 2002. *National survey of physicians part I: Doctors on disparities in medical care*. San Francisco, CA: Kaiser Family Foundation.

Kelley, A. S., and E. Bollens-Lund. 2018. Identifying the population with serious illness: The "denominator" challenge. *Journal of Palliative Medicine* 21:S-7–S-16.

Kerensky, T., and A. Y. Walley. 2017. Opioid overdose prevention and naloxone rescue kits: What we know and what we don't know. *Addiction Science & Clinical Practice* 12:4.

Kertesz, S., and A. J. Gordon. 2018. A crisis of opioids and the limits of prescription control: United States. *Addiction* 114(1):169–180.

Koyyalagunta, D., E. Bruera, C. Aigner, H. Nusrat, L. Driver, and D. Novy. 2013. Risk stratification of opioid misuse among patients with cancer pain using the SOAPP-SF. *Pain Medicine* 14(5):667–675.

Krane, E. J., S. J. Weisman, and G. A. Walco. 2018. The national opioid epidemic and the risk of outpatient opioids in children. *Pediatrics* 142(2):e20181623.

Larochelle, M. R., D. Bernson, T. Land, T. J. Stopka, N. Wang, Z. Xuan, S. M. Bagley, J. M. Liebschutz, and A. Y. Walley. 2018. Medication for opioid use disorder after nonfatal opioid overdose and association with mortality: A cohort study. *Annals of Internal Medicine* 169(3):137–145.

Lewis, M. 2018. Brain change in addiction as learning, not disease. *New England Journal of Medicine* 379(16):1551–1560.

Ma, J. D., J. M. Horton, M. Hwang, R. S. Atayee, and E. J. Roeland. 2014. A single-center, retrospective analysis evaluating the utilization of the opioid risk tool in opioid-treated cancer patients. *Journal of Pain & Palliative Care Pharmacotherapy* 28(1):4–9.

Marks, R. M., and E. J. Sachar. 1973. Undertreatment of medical inpatients with narcotic analgesics. *Annals of Internal Medicine* 78(2):173–181.

McCabe, S. E., C. J. Boyd, and A. Young. 2007. Medical and nonmedical use of prescription drugs among secondary school students. *Journal of Adolescent Health* 40(1):76–83.

McCabe, S. E., B. T. West, and C. J. Boyd. 2013. Medical use, medical misuse, and nonmedical use of prescription opioids: Results from a longitudinal study. *Pain* 154(5):708–713.

McCabe, S. E., P. Veliz, and J. E. Schulenberg. 2016. Adolescent context of exposure to prescription opioids and substance use disorder symptoms at age 35: A national longitudinal study. *Pain* 157(10):2173–2178.

Meghani, S. H. 2016. Intended target of the Centers for Disease Control and Prevention opioid guidelines. *JAMA Oncology* 2(9):1243.

Meghani, S. H., E. Byun, and R. M. Gallagher. 2012. Time to take stock: A meta-analysis and systematic review of analgesic treatment disparities for pain in the United States. *Pain Medicine* 13(2):150–174.

Merlin, J., S. R. Young, J. L. Starrels, S. Azari, E. J. Edelman, J. Pomeranz, P. Roy, S. Saini, W. C. Becker, and J. M. Liebschutz. 2018. Managing concerning behaviors in patients prescribed opioids for chronic pain: A Delphi study. *Journal of General Internal Medicine* 33(2):166–176.

Merlin, J. S., K. Patel, N. Thompson, J. Kapo, F. Keefe, J. Liebschutz, J. Paice, T. Somers, J. Starrels, J. Childers, Y. Schenker, and C. S. Ritchie. 2019. Managing chronic pain in cancer survivors prescribed long-term opioid therapy: A national survey of ambulatory palliative care providers. *Journal of Pain and Symptom Management* 57(1):20–27.

Miech, R., L. Johnston, P. M. O'Malley, K. M. Keyes, and K. Heard. 2015. Prescription opioids in adolescence and future opioid misuse. *Pediatrics* 136(5):e1169–e1177.

Morrison, R. S., S. Wallenstein, D. K. Natale, R. S. Senzel, and L. L. Huang. 2000. "We don't carry that"—failure of pharmacies in predominantly nonwhite neighborhoods to stock opioid analgesics. *New England Journal of Medicine* 342(14):1023–1026.

NAABT (National Alliance of Advocates for Buprenorphine Treatment). 2016. *What's this agonist/antagonist stuff?* https://www.naabt.org/faq_answers.cfm?ID=5 (accessed March 4, 2019).

NASEM (National Academies of Sciences, Engineering, and Medicine). 2019. *Medications for opioid use disorder save lives*. Washington, DC: The National Academies Press.

NCSL (National Conference of State Legislatures). 2018. *Prescribing policies: States confront opioid overdose epidemic*. http://www.ncsl.org/research/health/prescribing-policies-states-confront-opioid-overdose-epidemic.aspx (accessed March 19, 2019).

NIDA (National Institute on Drug Abuse). 2017. *Past-year misuse of prescription/over-the-counter vs. illicit drugs*. https://www.drugabuse.gov/related-topics/trends-statistics/infographics/monitoring-future-2017-survey-results (accessed March 5, 2019).

NIDA. 2019. *Overdose death rates*. https://www.drugabuse.gov/related-topics/trends-statistics/overdose-death-rates (accessed February 22, 2019).

Nikanne, E., H. Kokki, and K. Tuovinen. 1999. Postoperative pain after adenoidectomy in children. *British Journal Anaesthesia* 82(6):886–889.

Nixon, R. D., T. J. Nehmy, A. A. Ellis, S. A. Ball, A. Menne, and A. C. McKinnon. 2010. Predictors of posttraumatic stress in children following injury: The influence of appraisals, heart rate, and morphine use. *Behaviour Research and Therapy* 48(8):810–815.

Oliva, E., T. Bowe, S. Tavakoli, S. Martins, E. T. Lewis, M. Paik, I. Wiechers, P. Henderson, M. Harvey, T. Avoundjian, A. Medhanie, and J. A. Trafton. 2017. Development and applications of the Veterans Health Administration's Stratification Tool for Opioid Risk Mitigation (STORM) to improve opioid safety and prevent overdose and suicide. *Psychological Services* 14(1):34–49.

Paice, J. A. 2018. Navigating cancer pain management in the midst of the opioid epidemic. *Oncology (Williston Park)* 32(8):386–390, 403.

Passik, S. D., and D. E. Theobald. 2000. Managing addiction in advanced cancer patients: Why bother? *Journal of Pain and Symptom Management* 19(3):229–234.

Paulozzi, L. J., C. M. Jones, K. A. Mack, and R. A. Rudd. 2011. Vital signs: Overdoses of prescription opioid pain relievers—United States, 1999–2008. *Morbidity and Mortality Weekly Report* 60(43):1487–1492.

Pitt, A. L., K. Humphreys, and M. L. Brandeau. 2018. Modeling health benefits and harms of public policy responses to the US opioid epidemic. *American Journal of Public Health* 108(10):1394–1400.

Porter, J., and H. Hick. 1980. Addiction rare in patients treated with narcotics. *New England Journal of Medicine* 302:123.

Rauenzahn, S., A. Sima, B. Cassel, D. Noreika, T. H. Gomez, L. Ryan, C. E. Wolf, L. Legakis, and E. Del Fabbro. 2017. Urine drug screen findings among ambulatory oncology patients in a supportive care clinic. *Supportive Care in Cancer* 25(6):1859–1864.

Rossen, L. M., B. Bastian, M. Warner, D. Khan, and Y. Chong. 2017. Drug poisoning mortality: United States, 1999–2016. *National Center for Health Statistics*. https://www.cdc.gov/nchs/data-visualization/drug-poisoning-mortality (accessed March 6, 2019).

Saloner, B., J. Levin, H.-Y. Chang, C. Jones, and G. C. Alexander. 2018. Changes in buprenorphine-naloxone and opioid pain reliever prescriptions after the Affordable Care Act Medicaid expansion. *JAMA Network Open* 1(4):e181588.

Samet, J. H., M. Botticelli, and M. Bharel. 2018. Methadone in primary care—one small step for Congress, one giant leap for addiction treatment. *New England Journal Medicine* 379(1):7–8.

SAMHSA (Substance Abuse and Mental Health Services Administration). 2018. *42 CFR part 2 confidentiality of substance use disorder patient records*. https://www.samhsa.gov/health-information-technology/laws-regulations-guidelines (accessed February 26, 2019).

Saxe, G., F. Stoddard, D. Courtney, K. Cunningham, N. Chawla, R. Sheridan, D. King, and L. King. 2001. Relationship between acute morphine and the course of PTSD in children with burns. *Journal of the American Academy of Child & Adolescent Psychiatry* 40(8):915–921.

Schechter, N. L., D. A. Allen, and K. Hanson. 1986. Status of pediatric pain control: A comparison of hospital analgesic usage in children and adults. *Pediatrics* 77(1):11–15.

Schenker, Y., J. S. Merlin, and T. E. Quill. 2018. Use of palliative care earlier in the disease course in the context of the opioid epidemic: Educational, research, and policy issues. *JAMA* 320(9):871–872.

Scommegna, P. 2012. *More U.S. children raised by grandparents*. https://www.prb.org/us-children-grandparents (accessed March 4, 2019).

Skelly, A. C., R. Chour, J. R. Dettori, J. A. Turner, J. L. Friedly, S. D. Rundell, R. Fu, E. D. Brodt, N. Wasson, C. Winter, and A. J. R. Ferguson. 2018. *Noninvasive nonpharmacological treatment for chronic pain: A systematic review.* Rockville, MD: Agency for Healthcare Research and Quality.

Sordo, L., G. Barrio, M. J. Bravo, B. I. Indave, L. Degenhardt, L. Wiessing, M. Ferri, and R. Pastor-Barriuso. 2017. Mortality risk during and after opioid substitution treatment: Systematic review and meta-analysis of cohort studies. *BMJ* 357:j1550.

Staton, L. J., M. Panda, I. Chen, I. Genao, J. Kurz, M. Pasanen, A. J. Mechaber, M. Menon, J. O'Rorke, J. Wood, E. Rosenberg, C. Faeslis, T. Carey, D. Calleson, and S. Cykert. 2007. When race matters: Disagreement in pain perception between patients and their physicians in primary care. *Journal of the National Medical Association* 99(5):532–538.

Stoddard, F. J., Jr., E. A. Sorrentino, T. A. Ceranoglu, G. Saxe, J. M. Murphy, J. E. Drake, H. Ronfeldt, G. W. White, J. Kagan, N. Snidman, R. L. Sheridan, and R. G. Tompkins. 2009. Preliminary evidence for the effects of morphine on posttraumatic stress disorder symptoms in one- to four-year-olds with burns. *Journal of Burn Care & Research* 30(5):836–843.

Stover, M. W., and J. M. Davis. 2015. Opioids in pregnancy and neonatal abstinence syndrome. *Seminars in Perinatology* 39(7):561–565.

Tan, P. D., J. S. Barclay, and L. J. Blackhall. 2015. Do palliative care clinics screen for substance abuse and diversion? Results of a national survey. *Journal of Palliative Medicine* 18(9):752–757.

Umer, A., S. Loudin, S. Maxwell, C. Lilly, M. E. Stabler, L. Cottrell, C. Hamilton, J. Breyel, C. Mullins, and C. John. 2018. Capturing the statewide incidence of neonatal abstinence syndrome in real time: The West Virginia experience. *Pediatric Research* 85(5):607–611.

Unger, D. N. 2017. Pain medication & regulation: It is personal. *Journal of General Internal Medicine* 32(2):228–229.

U.S. Census Bureau. 2014. *Pop2 children as a percentage of the population: Persons in selected age groups as a percentage of the total U.S. population, and children ages 0–17 as a percentage of the dependent population, 1950–2017 and projected 2018–2050.* https://www.childstats.gov/americaschildren/tables/pop2.asp (accessed February 13, 2019).

Venkataramani, A. S., and P. Chatterjee. 2019. Early Medicaid expansions and drug overdose mortality in the USA: A quasi-experimental analysis. *Journal of General Internal Medicine* 34(1):23–25.

Volkow, N. D., G. F. Koob, and A. T. McLellan. 2016. Neurobiologic advances from the brain disease model of addiction. *New England Journal of Medicine* 374(4):363–371.

Weisman, S. J., B. Bernstein, and N. L. Schechter. 1998. Consequences of inadequate analgesia during painful procedures in children. *Archives of Pediatrics and Adolescent Medicine* 152(2):147–149.

Weiss, R. D., J. S. Potter, D. A. Fiellin, M. Byrne, H. S. Connery, W. Dickinson, J. Gardin, M. L. Griffin, M. N. Gourevitch, D. L. Haller, A. L. Hasson, Z. Huang, P. Jacobs, A. S. Kosinski, R. Lindblad, E. F. McCance-Katz, S. E. Provost, J. Selzer, E. C. Somoza, S. C. Sonne, and W. Ling. 2011. Adjunctive counseling during brief and extended buprenorphine-naloxone treatment for prescription opioid dependence: A 2-phase randomized controlled trial. *Archives of General Psychiatry* 68(12):1238–1246.

Wen, H., B. R. Schackman, B. Aden, and Y. Bao. 2017. States with prescription drug monitoring mandates saw a reduction in opioids prescribed to Medicaid enrollees. *Health Affairs (Millwood)* 36(4):733–741.

Wolfe, J., L. Orellana, C. Ullrich, E. F. Cook, T. I. Kang, A. Rosenberg, R. Geyer, C. Feudtner, and V. Dussel. 2015. Symptoms and distress in children with advanced cancer: Prospective patient-reported outcomes from the PediQUEST study. *Journal of Clinical Oncology* 33(17):1928–1935.

Yennurajalingam, S., T. Edwards, J. A. Arthur, Z. Lu, J. Najera, K. Nguyen, J. Manju, L. Kuriakose, J. Wu, D. Liu, J. L. Williams, S. K. Reddy, and E. Bruera. 2018. Predicting the risk for aberrant opioid use behavior in patients receiving outpatient supportive care consultation at a comprehensive cancer center. *Cancer* 124(19):3942–3949.

Appendix A

Statement of Task

An ad hoc committee will plan and host a 1-day workshop to examine ways to best address the pain management needs of people with serious illness in the context of widespread opioid use disorder, including consideration of the underlying socioeconomic factors that contribute to the epidemic. The workshop will feature invited presentations and panel discussions on topics that may include

- The Patient/Family Perspective
    - Impact of limitations in access to opioids on those with serious illness and their caregivers
    - Disparities in access to prescribed opioids for people with serious illness
    - Options for safe removal and disposal of opioids when they are no longer needed
- The Clinician Perspective
    - How restrictions on opioid prescribing affect clinicians and their ability to provide high-quality care for those with serious illness
    - Ways in which clinicians manage the care of seriously ill patients who have comorbid conditions such as cancer and substance use disorder

- The Payer Perspective
  - Challenges of striking a balance between access to opioid medications for patients' pain management and patient safety and prevention of opioid use disorder
- The Legislative/Policy Perspective
  - Potential impact of regulatory/legislative actions to address the opioid epidemic
  - Measures to protect the population of people with serious illness whose pain can only be effectively addressed by opioids
- Strategies to address gaps in the evidence base on pain management for people with serious illness

The committee will develop the agenda for the workshop, select speakers and discussants, and moderate the discussions. Proceedings of the presentations and discussions at the workshop will be prepared by a designated rapporteur in accordance with institutional guidelines.

Appendix B

Workshop Agenda

THURSDAY, NOVEMBER 29, 2018

8:00 am   **Registration and Breakfast**

8:30 am   **Welcome from the Roundtable on Quality Care for People with Serious Illness**
Leonard D. Schaeffer, University of Southern California (*Chair*) and
James Tulsky, M.D., Harvard Medical School (*Vice Chair*)

                Overview of the Workshop
Andrew Dreyfus, President and Chief Executive Officer, Blue Cross Blue Shield of Massachusetts and
James Tulsky, M.D., Chair, Department of Psychosocial Oncology and Palliative Care, Dana-Farber Cancer Institute; Chief, Division of Palliative Medicine, Brigham and Women's Hospital; Professor of Medicine and Co-Director, Center for Palliative Care, Harvard Medical School
Workshop Planning Committee Co-Chairs

8:40 am   **Session One: Understanding the Opioid Use Disorder Epidemic and Its Impact on Patients, Families, and Communities**

Introductory Video
Laura Martin, Substance Use Prevention Coordinator, City of Quincy, Massachusetts

Speaker:
— Jane Liebschutz, M.D., M.P.H., FACP, Chief, Division of General Internal Medicine, Professor of Medicine, Department of Medicine, University of Pittsburgh Medical Center (*@liebschutz / @PittGIM*)

9:10 am **Session Two: Pain Management for People with Serious Illness: Challenges and Opportunities in the Context of the Opioid Use Disorder Epidemic**

Moderator: R. Sean Morrison, M.D., Ellen and Howard C. Katz Professor, and Chair, Brookdale Department of Geriatrics and Palliative Medicine, Icahn School of Medicine at Mount Sinai

Patient and Caregiver Perspective: Ora Chaikin, Patient Voice, and
Rosanne Leipzig, M.D., Ph.D., Gerald and May Ellen Ritter Professor, Brookdale Department of Geriatrics and Palliative Medicine, Icahn School of Medicine at Mount Sinai

Speakers:
— Stefan Kertesz, M.D., M.Sc., Professor, Division of Preventive Medicine, University of Alabama at Birmingham School of Medicine (*@StefanKertesz*)
— Cardinale Smith, M.D., Ph.D., Associate Professor of Medicine, Director of Quality for Cancer Services, Mount Sinai Health System, Division of Hematology/Medical Oncology and Brookdale Department of Geriatrics and Palliative Medicine, Icahn School of Medicine at Mount Sinai (*@cardismith*)
— Stefan Friedrichsdorf, M.D., Medical Director, Department of Pain Medicine, Palliative Care & Integrative Medicine, Children's Hospitals and Clinics of Minnesota, University of Minnesota (*@NoNeedlessPain / @ChildrensMN*)

APPENDIX B   81

              Audience Q & A

11:00 am   Break

11:15 am   **Session Three: Addressing the Challenge of Patients with Comorbid Substance Use Disorder and Serious Illness**

Moderator: Judith Paice, Ph.D., R.N., Director, Cancer Pain Program, Division of Hematology-Oncology, and Research Professor of Medicine, Feinberg School of Medicine, Northwestern University (@LurieCancer)

Patient and Clinician Experience (videotaped discussion)— Patient and Dan Gorman, FNP-C, MSN, OCN, Director, Palliative Care Clinic, Dana-Farber Cancer Institute

Speaker:
— Jessica S. Merlin, M.D., Ph.D., M.B.A., Visiting Associate Professor of Medicine, Division of General Internal Medicine, Section of Palliative Care and Medical Ethics; Section of Treatment, Research, and Education in Addiction Medicine; Division of Infectious Diseases, University of Pittsburgh (*@JessicaMerlinMD / @PittGIM*)

Audience Q & A

12:15 pm   Lunch

1:15 pm   **Session Four: Impact of Policy and Regulatory Responses to the Opioid Use Disorder Epidemic on the Care of People with Serious Illness**

Moderator: James Tulsky, M.D., Chair, Department of Psychosocial Oncology and Palliative Care, Dana Farber Cancer Institute; Chief, Division of Palliative Medicine, Brigham and Women's Hospital; Professor of Medicine and Co-Director, Center for Palliative Care, Harvard Medical School (@jatulsky / @DanaFarber / @HMSPallCare)

Speakers:
- Hemi Tewarson, J.D., M.P.H., Division Director, Health Division, National Governors Association
- Michael Botticelli, M.Ed., Executive Director, Grayken Center for Addiction Medicine, Boston Medical Center, Former Director of National Drug Control Policy (*@MBotticelliBMC / @The_BMC*)
- Trent Haywood, M.D., J.D., Senior Vice President and Chief Medical Officer, Office of Clinical Affairs, Blue Cross Blue Shield Association

Audience Q & A

2:30 pm   **Break**

2:45 pm   **Session Five: Caring for People with Serious Illness in the Context of the Opioid Use Disorder Epidemic: Lessons to Inform Policy and Practice**

Moderator: Andrew Dreyfus, President and Chief Executive Officer, Blue Cross Blue Shield of Massachusetts (@andrewdreyfus / @BCBSMA)

Speakers:
- Bob Twillman, Ph.D., FACLP, Executive Director, Academy of Integrative Pain Management and Clinical Associate Professor, University of Kansas School of Medicine (*@BobTwillman / @TeamPainCare*)
- Jessica Nickel, Founder, President, and Chief Executive Officer, Addiction Policy Forum (*@jess_nickel / @AddictionPolicy*)
- Daniel Alford, M.D., M.P.H., Professor of Medicine, Associate Dean of Continuing Medical Education, Director, Clinical Addiction Research and Education (CARE) Unit, Director, Safe and Competent Opioid Prescribing Education (SCOPE of Pain) Program, Boston University School of Medicine Boston Medical Center (*@BUMedicine / @the_bmc*)

— Patrice Harris, M.D., M.A., President-Elect, American Medical Association, and Adjunct Professor, Department of Psychiatry and Behavioral Sciences, Emory University (*@AmerMedicalAssn*)
— Keith Humphreys, Ph.D., Esther Ting Memorial Professor, Psychiatry and Behavioral Sciences, Stanford University, and Senior Research Career Scientist, U.S. Department of Veterans Affairs (*@KeithNHumphreys*)

Audience Q & A

4:30 pm   **Closing Remarks**

4:35 pm   **Adjourn**